A HIGHER LOVE

A JOURNEY THROUGH ADDICTION, CANNABIS-INDUCED PSYCHOSIS, SUICIDE AND REDEMPTION

HEATHER BACCHUS

Copyright © 2024 Heather Bacchus

All rights reserved. No part of this publication may be reproduced or transmitted in any form or by any means, electronic or mechanical, including photocopy, recording, or any information storage and retrieval system, without permission in writing from the publisher.

The resources in this book are provided for informational purposes only and should not be used to replace the specialized training and professional judgment of a health care or mental health care professional.

Cover and book design by Asya Blue Design.

ISBN 979-8-9914654-0-3 Paperback
ISBN 979-8-9914654-1-0 Ebook

CONTENTS

Foreword 1

Introduction 5

Chapter 1: First Love 9

Chapter 2: Young Love 13

Chapter 3: Complex Love 19

Chapter 4: Turbulent Love 35

Chapter 5: Tough Love 49

Chapter 6: Love of Freedom 63

Chapter 7: Hopeful Love 75

Chapter 8: Helpless and Heartbreaking Love 89

Chapter 9: Unconditional Love 101

Chapter 10: Desperate Love 119

Chapter 11: Persistent Love 133

Chapter 12: Forgiving Love 147

Chapter 13: The Grief of Love................... 153

Chapter 14: Goodbye, My Love................. 161

Chapter 15: Love of Science 173

Chapter 16 : Love of Our Children 183

Epilogue: Love Remains 193

The Mystery.................................. 219

Signs of Cannabis Use......................... 221

Signs of Suicidal Behavior...................... 223

Acknowledgments 227

Index.. 231

FOREWORD

This generation faces a defining moment, not unlike the one faced by the Israelites in the valley of Elah. Then, with armies gathered around, a giant named Goliath mocked the army and demanded their best warrior to prove himself before him. For days, he challenged them. Each time, no one dared to rise and defeat him. Until a young shepherd named David, visiting his brothers, rose with faith and bravery, faced Goliath despite his mockery, and beat him, securing a historic victory for his people.

Now, as then, the juggernaut that is the marijuana industry and the societal acceptance they have relentlessly marketed to obtain bellows forth to America – daring us to challenge its lies and to do something about the lives it harms.

Now, as then, we wait for those deemed small in the eyes of this "Goliath" industry to rise to the occasion and defend our youth and every human's innate potential to live a truly free life.

This wait has been costly to my dear friends, Randy and Heather Bacchus. Their story of loss, love, and, ultimately, redemption could have been avoided. This wait has been costly to my dear friends Laura and Johnny Stack, whose story is similar in too many tragic ways. This wait has also been costly to the American people. As I write these words, the 2023 National Survey on Drug Use and Health (NSDUH), a federal survey of thousands of Americans, estimates more than 1.2 million youth meet the criteria for marijuana addiction. For young adults (18-25), this number expands to 5.6 million.

Millions of our nation's next generation are already dependent on marijuana, and the multi-billion dollar industry behind it has dramatically altered and made it more harmful. Do not fool yourself into reducing the words on the ensuing pages to a cautionary tale of low statistical probability. The facts of the Bacchus' story are not extreme or rare. The National Institute of Health supplied data in 2023 estimating that marijuana use is the primary factor in at least 30% of cases of schizophrenia among young men. Research published in the *Lancet Journal of Psychiatry* on these new, highly potent products also found regular use increases the probability of developing psychosis or schizophrenia more than five-fold.

Yes, Big Marijuana has hoodwinked our kids. Under the guise of a clever campaign to cloak their products in sheep's clothing, they changed the drug so fundamentally that science and public health are only now beginning to catch up – let alone public education – and our next generation is paying the price. Where did they learn to do this? We now know Altria, the former name for Phillip Morris, the largest tobacco company in America, has invested billions of dollars into marijuana. Other tobacco companies have followed suit, as well as Big Alcohol and a former executive from Purdue Pharma.

These industries lied to the American public and are responsible for the deaths of millions. They are using the 24 states as of this writing that legalized "recreational" marijuana and their billions in profits to unleash the same playbook again.

Returning to Elah, they rattle their sabers, mock parents, those with addiction, and the communities harmed. They lie to the public, saying their products are actually medicinal and not harmful. They bury the work of scientists attempting to reveal the truth and pay for biased research, undermining life-saving education for our children on today's marijuana. In short, Goliath awaits his challenger.

I have hope the wait may soon be over. You don't need to be a parent or have dependents to weep over the story of Randy Michael Bacchus. You don't need to have experience with the drug for you to grasp the tremendous harm marijuana can have, as it did in their lives. Enclosed, you will read one of the most authentic and vulnerable stories documenting what this substance can and is doing to families nationwide. Unlike opioids, sharing such a story is still widely mocked in the public sphere, and those raising their voices are written off.

Just like the young shepherd, David.

Randy and Heather have stepped out in faith, just as he did, to stand against the lies of this addiction-for-profit industry and the mass disinformation campaign that has kept the public asleep during this crisis. As so many of us gather along the battle lines, they have risen to defend our generation with all that they have, with their surviving children, to do what they can. Now, many more parents have answered their call and joined them, sharing their stories and courage.

For this reason, my organization, Smart Approaches to Marijuana (SAM), partnered with Texas Congressman Pete Sessions and U.S. Senator from Nebraska Pete Ricketts to introduce the bicameral (U.S. House and Senate) "Randy's Resolution," honoring his life and calling the nation to action on the dangers of high-potency marijuana.

In a country like America, parents *can* create generational change. This book represents the beginning of a change in the tide. I will stand beside them to speak out and fight for the next generation of young Americans being targeted by this industry.

Will you?

Luke Niforatos
Executive Vice President,
Smart Approaches to Marijuana (SAM)
Co-Founder, Foundation for Drug Policy Solutions (FDPS)

INTRODUCTION

On July 17, 2021, I woke up to a text message from our twenty-one-year-old son, Randy Michael: "I love you, Mom, and am sorry for everything. Please tell Dad the same. I wish I would have been a better person."

Just moments after sending that text, Randy Michael took his own life.

It breaks my heart that he died thinking he wasn't a good person. He was a good person, a truly remarkable soul. But he was addicted to marijuana, which he started using at a very young age. This potent, addictive product changed his developing brain, made him mentally ill, and led to his suicide.

Two months after Randy Michael's death, we received his computers and phones and soon realized that our son had left us an enormous gift of information and insights; what we found was a window into his mental state in the months before his untimely death.

Although Randy Michael usually appeared to function fairly well, his writings, photos, and videotapes revealed that he was succumbing to delusions, falling apart, and fading into a shadow of the person he had once been.

Until we saw his journals, vlogs, and photos, we had no idea how much he had been suffering—and no idea how much marijuana was affecting his downfall. In the last two years of his life in his private writings, Randy Michael exhibited paranoia, grandiosity, delusions, mania, suicidal ideation, anxiety, and depression. At the time, we did not understand how much marijuana was contributing to those problems.

Our son believed marijuana was medicine, and he frequently shared all the industry talking points about its benefits, especially if we criticized marijuana or questioned his use of it. We did not know then that there are more than twenty thousand scientific studies on the effects of marijuana that we could have used to challenge his assertions.

We know now. And I am writing this book to make sure others know too.

This book tells a love story—or many love stories, actually. It begins with a typical story of romance where girl meets boy and falls in love, but it moves on to explore vastly different types of love—and the pain that love can bring.

Our journey would eventually travel into the joy of loving three daughters and a son—and the nightmare of losing that beloved son to marijuana addiction. The truth is that we lost Randy Michael—and he lost himself—long before his final day.

Sadly, our journey has led us into a broader community of countless families like ours who have grappled with the loss of a loved one due to addiction. We have connected with others nationwide whose children have faced the consequences of modern-day marijuana use and heard many stories that all too closely resemble our family's story.

INTRODUCTION

More and more states are moving toward the legalization, commercialization, and normalization of cannabis usage, and as of 2024, almost half of US states allow the commercial sales of marijuana. The federal government is now also apparently considering changing marijuana's legal status. But these moves seem to be happening without decision-makers fully grappling with the reality that marijuana is a potent, intoxicating, addictive, and psychoactive drug or recognizing that the marijuana of today differs fundamentally from the substance of previous generations. Today's product is much stronger, comes in many different forms, is promoted to meet any daily need, and is often touted as medicinal.

I fear that many people already perceive marijuana as safe and more will follow suit as it becomes legal in more places, so I am writing this book because I want everyone to know this: *The marijuana of the 2020s is anything but safe.*

Many experts fear that the widespread use of today's marijuana products will lead to an increase in traffic violations, more fatal accidents from drivers under the influence, increasing and amplified mental health issues, suicidal ideation, and an uptick in violence and crime. And I fear that more families will face the problems my family has faced.

Kevin Sabet, author of the book *Smokescreen* and one of the founders of the nonprofit organization Smart Approaches to Marijuana, has said, "There isn't a problem that drugs can't make worse." Having lived with addiction, we know this is true.

My family is sharing our story so that readers can recognize the risks of high-potency marijuana products and hemp-derived psychoactive cannabis products to offer an alternative path. We share our story so that families facing similar struggles won't feel isolated or ashamed. We share our story so that we can describe signs that have given us hope and brought us healing after unimaginable loss.

Ultimately, we share our story because we want to help others avoid the tragic turn that has been written into our family's love story. By highlighting relevant scientific studies our goal is to help educate parents, young people, politicians, teachers, law enforcement, and first responders about the risks of today's high-potency marijuana to the developing brain. If we can prevent even one teen from experiencing the problems of drug use, we will have helped spare an entire family the chaos, uncertainty, pain, and loss that go hand in hand with addiction.

I want to provide the facts so that parents will know how to respond when their child confidently declares, "It's just weed—a nonaddictive plant, a natural substance, a medicine."

Because nothing could be further from the truth.

CHAPTER 1

FIRST LOVE

Marriage and Family

My husband, Randy, and I met in October 1990 at a bar in our college town. I was twenty, and he was twenty-one. We greeted each other briefly and then parted ways. I was extremely shy and had *never* asked out anyone, yet I had this overwhelming inclination to ask this boy I had barely met to go on a date with me.

Although I heard he had a girlfriend, I still asked if he wanted to go to a party with me. Of course, Randy said, "No, I have a girlfriend," but I continued to think about him.

A couple of months later, I found out they had broken up. So, I tried again, and this time he agreed to go to a movie with me.

From that first night, I knew I loved him. He was tall with remarkably dark hair, beautiful skin, captivating green eyes, and a smile that truly ensnared me. His humor resonated with me, and I instantly felt a desire to spend the rest of my life with him. While some may not believe in love at first sight, I certainly do.

Randy and I had both grown up in White Bear Lake, Minnesota, but our paths did not cross until college. I knew of him, though. In November 1986, a small plane crash killed Randy's mother, father, two brothers, and his sister in Steamboat, Colorado. A senior at a local Catholic high school, Randy had stayed home to study for finals. Devastatingly, his father was piloting the small plane that did not clear the mountain, and in an instant, their family of six became one. Our community was shaken by the tragic news, and I remember it vividly. I was a junior in a public high school at the time of the crash, and I remember feeling so sorry for this young man who had just lost his entire family. Although I didn't know him personally, I couldn't imagine surviving such a catastrophic loss.

When Randy and I met in college, I didn't immediately connect him with the crash, and he waited awhile to share the heartbreaking story with me. I never knew Randy's immediate family, but their absence and my husband's tragic loss have profoundly shaped our lives and our family. Because I have witnessed my husband struggle with this enormous loss, I hold immense respect for his resilience, faith, ability to love, and tenacity for life.

Randy and I dated on and off for about three years before we got married in 1995. I recall him looking at me during our grand wedding and saying, "This is one of my best days." It was also a very challenging day for Randy. The vase of five white roses on the altar could not make up for his absent family.

When we married, Randy was working as a Realtor, while I worked as a substitute elementary school teacher and as a sales associate at a department store. Eventually, Randy decided to carry on a family tradition and started a construction company to build single-family homes.

No Guarantees

As we celebrated our first wedding anniversary, I learned I was pregnant! Both of us were extremely excited to begin a family together. When I entered my second trimester, I became anxious about setting up the nursery. I was ready to paint the room, put up the crib, set up the rocking chair, and hang the mobile.

However, Randy did not share my enthusiasm. He said it was too early. He preferred to set up the nursery closer to our due date. "Just in case."

I voiced my frustration to my mom, who, with greater wisdom and insight than I had, gently reminded me that because of his life experiences, Randy knew nothing in life was guaranteed.

Eventually, the nursery was ready by the time Brooke was born in August 1997. I so enjoyed motherhood that I decided to leave teaching and sales and commit to raising our family day in and day out. In November 1999, Brooke became a proud big sister to Randy Michael. In January 2002, Sabrina was born, followed by Anna in September 2004.

After every birth, my mom and dad, my siblings and their spouses, and my nieces and nephews all came to the hospital to greet their newest family member. On occasions like that, Randy's missing immediate family loomed large.

Of course, Randy enjoyed his loving aunts, uncles, and teenage cousins, but his nuclear family has been missing from every single special event of his life since he was seventeen. I always tried to be thoughtful about that absence, but I did not truly understand his loss.

As our family grew, I felt like those absences became less noticeable, although they have never been forgotten. Randy chose to move forward despite his great void, and our family was filled with love, activity, and joy. We cherished family vacations, enjoyed memorable moments on White Bear Lake, and treasured time with family and friends. We attended Mass regularly, read books, played sports, shared family dinners, enrolled our kids in the best schools, took them for regular doctor visits, and did everything possible to raise happy, healthy children.

Yet, tragically, I would eventually come to personally experience a sense of my husband's loss. I learned how hard it is to navigate an absence. I found out firsthand about navigating loss and grief.

And I have come to the undeniable understanding that Randy was right: nothing in life is guaranteed.

CHAPTER 2

YOUNG LOVE

Randy Michael's Early Years

Randy Michael was born on November 9, 1999. A Paul Bunyan–sized baby at nine pounds, three ounces, he arrived with beautiful hands and long fingers, but not a single hair on his head! As a newborn, he was a sleepy, laid-back soul, and I loved to watch as his fingers lazily played in the air. I had to gently tickle his feet and unzip his sleeper just to rouse him enough to feed him.

When he was three months old, we traveled to visit his grandparents in Florida, and the trip seemed to ignite a change in him. The warmth and radiance of the sunshine seemed to stir his spirit, and he began eating heartily and growing swiftly, tipping the scales at twenty-eight pounds by his first birthday.

A delightful and easygoing baby, Randy Michael shared a special bond with his sister, Brooke, as he began to crawl and string together his first words. They were constant companions and playmates. By the time he was sixteen months old, he was walking, beginning to talk, and displaying his social personality.

Sabrina was born shortly after Randy Michael's second birthday. He enjoyed being a big brother, gently holding the baby and calling her "Sabeweena" in a deep, raspy voice. Always entertaining, his playful antics never failed to elicit giggles from Sabrina. During their early years, the two of them always kept me on my toes.

When he was about two and a half, he started having trouble sleeping. We suspected enlarged tonsils but removing them did not alleviate his sleeping issues. His night terrors persisted, and his behavior became increasingly impulsive.

Randy Michael started attending a Montessori school shortly before his fourth birthday. Although he coped reasonably well, he seemed to often feel overwhelmed by the variety of activities that were offered. He spent many days/hours at school "walking the line," stepping back and forth on a line until he could decide on what activity to start.

Tics and Terrors

Anna was born in September, shortly before Randy Michael's fifth birthday. He was a kind and loving big brother, but because of his persistent night terrors, increasingly impulsive behavior, and a lack of focus at school, we scheduled an evaluation at Children's Hospital in St. Paul, Minnesota, when he was five-and-a-half years old. It was determined he had a tic disorder, which is marked by irregular, uncontrollable, and repetitive movements of muscles that can occur in any part of the body. The tics can be motor or vocal. We knew that Randy Michael exhibited a vocal snorting tic, but we had not realized that he also had a motor tic that involved an eye muscle.

As a young and busy mom, I was upset about this diagnosis,

of course, but it also frustrated me because the tics did not seem that significant. I was much more concerned by his temper tantrums, impulsive behavior, hyperactivity, and persistent night terrors, which we believed were affecting his daily behavior because they interrupted his sleep.

After consulting with his doctor, a child psychologist, and the Montessori school teacher, the professionals added attention deficit hyperactivity disorder (ADHD) in addition to his tic disorder. We opted to start medication for his ADHD when Randy Michael was six years old. The first medication he took was Concerta, and his Montessori teacher for the previous two years noticed a significant transformation—like witnessing a whole new kid! As Randy Michael became more focused and better at selecting and completing tasks, he enjoyed a fantastic and successful kindergarten year.

At his "fly up" ceremony marking the end of kindergarten, our six-year-old son stood in front of a room filled with parents and grandparents and confidently reported on knights and dished out math facts to his peers. Social and engaging, Randy Michael clearly enjoyed all the attention. Despite lingering sleep issues, his school focus had improved, and he had cultivated better relationships with his sisters at home. We were grateful for these strides!

Elementary School Challenges

Randy Michael began first grade at a small Catholic school near our home in White Bear Lake. An early start time at the school made for challenging mornings around our house, while fights over his homework made for some rough afternoons and evenings. As the year went on, signs of dyslexia emerged.

He was still suffering from sleep issues, so Randy Michael underwent evaluations with a sleep doctor. After they ruled out seizures or neurological disorders, the doctor prescribed medication for the sleep terrors. His sleeping patterns improved, and we were hopeful.

We moved in 2007 to a neighboring community—Mahtomedi, Minnesota—when Randy Michael was in second grade and enrolled the kids in another small Catholic school. This school had a much more reasonable start time, especially for a child with sleep issues, and made it easier to get four small children out the door well-rested and content.

But Randy Michael continued to struggle with reading and was also grappling with dysgraphia—consistently writing in mirror images—tendencies that dated back to his Montessori days. Our concerns about his learning skills intensified, prompting an evaluation from our local school district, which concluded that Randy Michael continued to struggle with ADHD, mild dyslexia, slow processing speed, and challenges with executive functioning skills. On the bright side, he had the memorization capabilities of a sixteen-year-old at the age of seven.

We collaborated closely with Randy Michael's teachers to address these challenges, continuing the use of Concerta, and adding therapy sessions to tackle behavioral and sensory issues. Over time, these interventions resulted in tangible improvements for Randy Michael in his academic and social pursuits.

With Randy Michael making commendable strides in school, life at home found a more peaceful rhythm, and we were hopeful that the progress would continue. But the smooth trajectory became rocky again when he was in sixth grade.

As Randy Michael's academic performance began declining, he adopted a class-clown persona and occasionally landed in trouble for bullying other students. After each incident, we implemented consequences at home, facilitated apologies to those affected, and engaged in discussions about his behavior. After this tumultuous school year, we sought another psychological evaluation. Consistent with previous assessments, professionals confirmed that Randy Michael was challenged by ADHD, low executive functioning skills, and slow processing. However, they also highlighted his strengths, noting exceptional memorization abilities as well as strong verbal and written skills. The evaluation blamed Randy Michael's slipping grades on his slower processing speed, noting that he would need additional tutoring support to keep up as coursework became increasingly demanding.

Faced with the reality that Randy Michael was not prepared to enter seventh grade at his current school, we investigated making an expensive investment in private tutoring. But after doing more research, we decided to move him to our local Catholic middle and high school. This small, private school would provide him more access to individualized tutoring and other educational resources through its Learning Center, which specializes in working with students who have individualized education plans.

CHAPTER 3

COMPLEX LOVE

Navigating Early Adolescence

Randy Michael thrived when he moved to Hill-Murray. He loved the larger student body, and he participated in sports, explored art courses, improved his grades, and forged new friendships.

Two senior boys embraced Randy Michael and his friend "Aaron,"[1] taking them under their wings and mentoring them as they transitioned into a new school landscape. The seniors were on the hockey team and getting attention from these two high-status upperclassmen made the two seventh graders feel like rock stars. Randy Michael continued to flourish academically and socially through eighth grade.

Things changed when Randy Michael entered ninth grade. He smiled less and withdrew more, spending hours alone in his room. As his carefree demeanor waned, his grades began to drop off again, and we noticed he was spending less time with his familiar circle of friends and more with kids we didn't know as well.

---

[1] To protect some people's identity, I have renamed some individuals in this story. Those names appear in quote marks on first use.

Concerned, I reached out to other parents, wondering if they or their kids could shed any light on Randy Michael's new behavior, but no one offered us any insight. When I confronted Randy Michael directly, he reassured me that everything was fine and denied facing any new challenges.

With no evidence to the contrary, we attributed the changes in our son to typical teenage development patterns. Adolescents often pull away from their families as they seek greater independence. Their friends are changing too, so it's not unusual for teens to shuffle their social circles during the high school years. I remembered that my friends had changed when I was about Randy Michael's age, so I tried not to worry.

A Shattering Phone Call

But a phone call in the summer after Randy Michael's freshman year shattered any illusion that all was well. A friend called to say she had discovered that her son had been smoking marijuana and that Randy Michael had been involved with him. Snapchat conversations and texts showed our sons planning to buy marijuana once again from a local dealer. Randy Michael was just fifteen.

We confronted Randy Michael immediately and reminded him that our family was strongly opposed to any kind of drug use. We had witnessed the toll of addiction in our own families, so we never looked at drug use as a harmless teenage phase.

We took away Randy Michael's cell phone and grounded him for a week, and we tried to impress upon him the dangers associated with using marijuana, focusing on concerns about motivation and academic success. We certainly never wanted Randy Michael to become a burnout or stoner like the kids we had seen in our own high school days.

However, we didn't tell him that the marijuana he was using was far more potent than the weed our high school peers had passed around in the 1980s. We didn't tell him that because we didn't know about the difference in potency or how the current high-potency products could damage his young and developing mind.

You Need to Know

Cannabis is a genus of flowering plants. There are over three hundred different species, but the two types of plants most talked about are hemp and marijuana, which itself has two subtypes: indica and sativa. What's the difference? Indica tends to produce a more relaxing effect, and sativa tends to have a more energizing effect.

Legal hemp contains less than .3 percent tetrahydrocannabinol (THC or Delta-9), the psychoactive and intoxicating component of the plant that gets users high and has an abundance of cannabidiol (CBD). CBD is not intoxicating, yet it has been approved by the FDA for treating two rare childhood seizure disorders. This medication is called Epidiolex and is 100 percent pure CBD, and it does not contain any THC. Also, there is some anecdotal evidence that CBD can provide relief for acute bouts of anxiety (e.g., before public speaking) and some physical health problems.

CBD can be chemically altered to produce synthetic analogs of Delta-9-THC, such as Delta-8, Delta-10, THC-O, and THC-P. These cannabinoids, known as Hemp-derived psychoactive cannabinoids are created using a chemical process, some of which may involve harmful substances such as butane, propane, or ethanol. States have struggled to regulate the sale of these cannabinoids and it is important to note that Hemp-derived THC has the same negative impact on the developing brain as THC from marijuana posing risks to youth and adolescents.

Marijuana contains significantly more of the intoxicating THC and much less CBD than hemp does.

Today's marijuana products are much stronger than the marijuana that was around from the 1960s through the 1990s. The typical THC potency level of the product in the 1960s and 1970s was 1 percent THC; by the 1980s, potency had increased to around 3 percent; it rose to about 5 percent THC in the 1990s. Marijuana growers have genetically modified the plant and discovered the perfect growing conditions, increasing the potency over the decades. Today's marijuana potency, in just the flower alone, can go as high as 35 percent THC, not to mention that the concentrates can be up to 95 percent THC.[2] Using a product with a higher potency increases the likelihood of developing a cannabis use disorder.[3]

Different Forms of Marijuana and Their Consumption Methods

Smokable Flower

Smoking the bud from the plant produces effects almost immediately. Marijuana smokers consume the flower using the following methods:

- **Joint:** Also known as a cannabis or marijuana cigarette, a joint consists of ground marijuana flower rolled in paper and smoked.

- **Blunt:** Like a joint, a blunt uses a blunt wrap or an emptied cigar to hold the ground flower.

---

2 E. B. Stuyt, "The Problem with the Current High Potency THC Marijuana from the Perspective of an Addiction Psychiatrist," *Missouri Medicine* 115, no. 6 (2018): 482–86, https://pubmed.ncbi.nlm.nih.gov/30643324.

3 Kat Petrilli, Shelan Ofori, Lindsey Hines, Gemma Taylor, Sally Adams, and Tom P. Freeman, "Association of Cannabis Potency with Mental Ill Health and Addiction: A Systematic Review," *The Lancet Psychiatry* 9, no. 9 (2022): 736–50, https://doi.org/10.1016/s2215-0366(22)00161-4.

- **Pipe:** Ground flower is placed in a pipe, lit up, and smoked, eliminating the need for rolling papers or blunts.

- **Bong:** A bong, or water pipe, filters the smoke through water for a milder inhalation experience.

Dabbing

Dabbing is a method of consuming concentrated forms of cannabis, known as dabs. Dabs are potent doses of cannabis made by extracting THC and other cannabinoids using a solvent like butane or CO_2. The resulting products—such as wax, shatter, oil, or budder—are named after their consistency and have a high THC concentration, often ranging from 60 to 95 percent. Dabbing is an extremely potent high and effects are felt immediately.

How Does Dabbing Work?

- **Preparation:** A small amount of the concentrate (dab) is placed on a dab tool.

- **Heating:** A dab rig, which resembles a traditional bong, is equipped with a "nail" made of glass, quartz, ceramic, or titanium. The nail is heated using a torch until it is red hot.

- **Application:** Once the nail reaches the desired temperature, the dab is applied to the hot surface.

- **Inhalation:** As the concentrate vaporizes upon contact with the hot nail, the user inhales the vapor through the mouthpiece of the rig.

Vaping

Vaping THC involves inhaling vaporized THC. It is gaining in popularity due to its discreteness, ease of use, and perceived health benefits compared to traditional smoking.

Vape concentrates can range between 30 and 90 percent THC. Effects are felt immediately. Youth will often say their vaping cartridge is "just nicotine," but there is no way to tell without looking at the vape cartridge that is inserted into the device.

How Does Vaping THC Work?

- **Devices:** THC is vaped using various devices, such as vape pens, portable vaporizers, and desktop vaporizers. They can be reusable or disposable and disguised to look like ordinary products. Examples are a highlighter, a pen, or even a water bottle where the straw is actually the device.

- **Forms:** The THC can be in different forms, including THC oil, distillate, or dry herb.

- **Heating:** The device heats the THC product to a temperature that is high enough to vaporize the active compounds without combustion.

- **Inhalation:** The user inhales the vapor, delivering THC to the bloodstream through the lungs.

THC Edibles

THC edibles are food and drink products that are infused with tetrahydrocannabinol (THC). An alternative to smoking or vaping, edibles allow users to consume discreetly and with longer-lasting effects.

The serving size in Colorado is ten milligrams, but a candy, cookie, or edible product may contain anywhere from five milligrams or more of THC. As a result, a serving could be a fourth of a candy, depending on how many milligrams of THC it contains.

Types of THC Edibles

- **Baked goods:** Brownies, cookies, cakes, and other pastries infused with THC.
- **Candies:** Gummies, lollipops, chocolates, and hard candies containing THC.
- **Beverages:** THC-infused drinks like sodas, teas, coffees, and alcoholic beverages.
- **Savory foods:** Infused snacks such as chips, popcorn, and baked goods.
- **Cooking ingredients:** THC-infused oils, butters, and tinctures that can be added to homemade dishes.

How THC Edibles Work

When THC is consumed in an edible form, it is metabolized differently compared to inhalation methods:

- **Ingestion:** The edible is eaten and the THC travels through the digestive system.
- **Metabolism:** THC is absorbed into the bloodstream through the stomach and intestines, and then processed by the liver. The liver converts THC into 11-hydroxy-THC, a potent metabolite.
- **Onset:** Effects typically take longer to begin, between thirty minutes to two hours, due to the digestive process.
- **Duration:** The effects of THC edibles can last much longer than those of inhaled THC, often four to twelve hours, depending on the dose and the user's individual metabolism.

Naively, we believed a lecture and some stern discipline would turn Randy Michael away from marijuana, but our son was not at all convinced by our explanations and advice. Instead, he adamantly argued that pot was harmless.

"It's natural and not addictive," he claimed, "just a plant, created by God."

He wholeheartedly embraced the industry's "pot propaganda," which downplays the dangers of marijuana while emphasizing its benefits and touting its "safety."

At the time, we didn't fully realize the source of the viewpoints that Randy Michael was embracing. Today, I believe that this misleading narrative is fostered by an industry driven by the love of profit, even if it comes at the expense of public health, truth, and well-being. A truly different kind of love, a selfish love: the love of a healthy bottom line!

Randy Michael stopped using for a little while, but by Christmas break during his sophomore year, he had started again. By the time spring rolled around, he was using marijuana regularly with school friends and neighborhood acquaintances. During his sophomore year, another one of Randy Michael's friend's mothers reached out to tell me she had found a kitchen scale in her son's backpack, supposedly for selling marijuana "just to friends." Our son was one of those friends.

I was shocked when the woman told me she occasionally permitted her son, "James," to smoke at home, claiming his doctor said it was "good for him" because he had sustained a brain injury a few years earlier. Although I had not fully grasped the dangers of marijuana on a developing brain at that time, I still found it bewildering that a doctor would say it was "good for him." And I wasn't amused when the mom made some sort of joke about how she might like to use marijuana herself from time to time. I knew her casual attitude didn't help our case.

James held the "cool kid" status at school, and his mother was the "cool mom," because she was okay with him using marijuana. Randy Michael was witnessing James smoke with his mother's blessing, even though he had suffered a brain injury. That further reinforced his ideas that pot was beneficial; my warnings to the contrary seemed silly to Randy Michael. In my heart, I knew marijuana wasn't good for these young men, but I wasn't armed then with the scientific studies that confirmed the risks.[4] Today, I have read many research studies that validate the concerns I felt at the time.[5]

> ### *You Need to Know*
>
> Addiction is frequently a pediatric-onset disorder, meaning that the overwhelming majority of individuals who develop a substance use disorder or an addiction—involving alcohol, nicotine, marijuana, opioids, cocaine, or any other substance—began using during their adolescent years. The risk of developing a substance-use disorder significantly escalates when individuals begin substance use before the age of twenty-one. Delaying the initiation of substance use of any kind in our youth can effectively reduce the likelihood of addiction later in life.[6]

---

4 Yasmin L. Hurd et al., "Cannabis and the Developing Brain: Insights into Its Long-Lasting Effects," *The Journal of Neuroscience* 39, no. 42 (2019): 8250–58, https://www.jneurosci.org/content/39/42/8250.

5 Joanna Jacobus and Susan F. Tapert, "Effects of Cannabis on the Adolescent Brain," *Current Pharmaceutical Design* 20, no. 13 (2014): 2186–93, https://doi.org/10.2174/13816128113199990426.

6 L. Searcy, "The Disease of Addiction: A Critical Pediatric Prevention Issue," *Journal of Pediatric Health Care* 31, no. 1 (2017): 2–4, https://doi.org/10.1016/j.pedhc.2016.10.001.

A Shattering Death

On April 21, 2016, I received a text from Aaron's mom. Aaron had been Randy Michael's close friend in grade school and middle school. "Liz" was writing to let me know that Aaron was dead. I read the text repeatedly to ensure that I had understood the message correctly. It felt surreal. It was a school holiday, so I rushed downstairs and woke Randy Michael to ask if Aaron had been sick. Rubbing the sleep from his eyes, unaware of Aaron's death, Randy Michael mumbled, "No, I think sometimes he gets stomachaches, but not that I know of."

Still in a state of disbelief and uncertain of what to do, I nervously dialed Liz. In a hushed tone, Liz answered the phone. The only thing I could think of to say was, "Liz, I am so sorry. What happened?"

Between gasps of breath and in a whisper of a voice, she explained that Aaron had died by suicide the night before. Suddenly, I felt the room swirling around me. I had assumed Aaron must have been battling an unknown physical ailment; never did I suspect that he had taken his own life. It was incomprehensible. Aaron was a sweet and kind soul who had been raised in a loving, supportive, and nurturing environment. He was tender, sensitive, and bright, and possessed a wonderful sense of humor. He was one of Randy Michael's only friends who had not been using drugs. However, he had been suffering silently with his sorrows and anxiety.

His impulsive and permanent decision shocked us all and left a profound impact on many. Our family and school community were shattered. I felt a weight on my chest, an ache in my stomach, and a fog in my head, and I knew my pain was only a shadow of what Aaron's family was feeling. The thought of never seeing Aaron's beautiful big eyes and smile again filled me with despair, and I worried about how his classmates and friends would handle it, especially Randy Michael.

Overwhelmed with disbelief and sorrow, yet bolstered by my husband's encouragement, Randy Michael and I rushed over to Aaron's home, carrying food and hoping to provide some solace. As we prepared to enter Aaron's home, I remembered an evening I had spent at Children's Hospital in St. Paul when Anna was about three months old and dealing with a bout of RSV. I heard a code called over the loudspeaker, and then heart-wrenching screams and moans reverberated through the halls. Our nurse entered our room to explain that a family in the neighboring room had just lost their three-year-old. This was the second child they had lost to a genetic condition. I couldn't help but weep, hearing the family express a pain I hoped to never know. I prayed for them as I sat beside my own child's bedside, grateful that Anna was going to be okay yet struggling with unanswerable questions. *Why? Why would these parents have to suffer through the loss of two children?* Those feelings of pain and shock and the questions came back to me as we stepped into Aaron's home.

Liz was stretched out on the sofa, engulfed in sobs, and grappling with an endless stream of questions. Her anguish was palpable as she embarked on the agonizing quest for answers—the pursuit of whys in the wake of this excruciating loss of her beautiful son. This process is all too familiar to us now, and one that lingers indefinitely.

After a heart-wrenching visit, we headed back home and pulled into the garage. Randy Michael's phone rang, and I could hear his friend James ask, "Hey, do you want to get high before the prayer service for Aaron?"

What did I just hear? I was shocked, afraid, and incredibly disappointed. With my head on a swivel, my eyes pivoted to Randy

Michael, and I suggested he hang up the phone. Randy Michael and I sat in the car and talked. He revealed that Aaron had tried to reach him the night before to invite him to game online, but he couldn't because he was out celebrating *420 Day* and getting high with James. Randy Michael called Aaron back after he got home around 9 p.m. There was no answer. Aaron was already gone.

Suddenly rage at Randy Michael and James overwhelmed my sadness. How could they even consider such a thing, especially after what had just happened the night before?

The situation left me angry, sad, and incredibly concerned. None of this felt acceptable or right. But while implementing consequences for Randy Michael's actions, we worried that he might feel a weight of responsibility for the loss. The complexity of the situation demanded unwavering vigilance, empathy, therapy, genuine concern, and prayer. Our priority was supporting Randy Michael through this devastating loss and convincing him to give up smoking weed.

While Randy Michael posed challenges, he was also a deeply compassionate, caring, and sensitive individual. He felt compelled to honor Aaron by writing a eulogy and dressing up for the service. The night before Aaron's service, I took our son shopping for a suit—he had grown nearly six inches in the past year! Randy Michael worked late into the night before the funeral, pouring his heart into crafting a tribute for his friend. We didn't read the eulogy before he delivered it. The next afternoon in front of classmates, teachers, and numerous families, Randy Michael eloquently expressed his affection and fondness for his dear friend Aaron and received many compliments for a job well done.

You Need to Know

What does 420 mean? Fifty years ago, 420 was a secret code among a small group of friends. It represented a time—4:20 p.m.—when this group would meet to smoke marijuana. Over time, 420 has morphed into a globally known holiday among cannabis lovers. Annually on April 20, cannabis users will gather at 4:20 p.m. to promote legalization, rally, and have concerts and parties, especially in legal-use states. This has become common knowledge in cannabis culture. Know the whereabouts of your child on this date if marijuana use is a concern and have a conversation about 420.

You Need to Know

Higher THC levels may mean a greater risk for addiction, especially if people are regularly exposing themselves to high doses.[7] It is clear to me now that even though Randy Michael had only been using marijuana for less than a year, it was a habit teetering on daily use and becoming an addiction.

For the first time in American history, the number of daily marijuana users has surpassed the number of daily alcohol users. In 2022, approximately 17.7 million people reported using marijuana on a daily or near daily basis, compared to 14.7 million daily or near daily drinkers.[8] As states have legalized and commercialized recreational marijuana, the perception of harm has gone down, and its use has escalated.[9]

---

7 National Institute on Drug Abuse, "Cannabis (Marijuana) DrugFacts," December 2019, https://nida.nih.gov/publications/drugfacts/cannabis-marijuana.

8 Jonathan P. Caulkins, "Changes in Self-Reported Cannabis Use in the United States from 1979 to 2022," *Addiction* (May 2024), https://doi.org/10.1111/add.16519.

9 Kathleen Gali, Sandra J. Winter, Naina J. Ahuja, Erica Frank, and Judith J. Prochaska, "Changes in Cannabis Use, Exposure, and Health Perceptions following Legalization of Adult Recreational Cannabis Use in California: A Prospective Observational Study," *Substance Abuse Treatment, Prevention, and Policy* 16, no. 1 (2021), https://doi.org/10.1186/s13011-021-00352-3.

Offering Support, Pursuing Accountability

Knowing how much Randy Michael would miss Aaron, we continued to offer our unwavering support and love by ensuring he received counseling and striving to be both gentle and patient. However, we also sought to maintain accountability and let our son know we would not allow him to use marijuana while living in our house.

We pursued professional guidance for Randy Michael, and my therapist recommended that he attend Wilderness Adventure Camp or an Outward-Bound program. However, he was reluctant, and his dad and I did not agree on the matter, adding another layer of challenge to our situation. After yet another incident early in the summer where Randy Michael snuck out of his bedroom in the dead of night, we settled on a compromise: he would volunteer at a Muscular Dystrophy Association (MDA) camp. For one week he would be responsible for one camper with muscular dystrophy. We hoped that caring for individuals facing physical challenges would cultivate a deeper appreciation for his own health and body and discourage him from further substance use.

Randy Michael wound up cherishing his time at the MDA camp so much that he returned to volunteer for two more summers. He formed strong bonds with the campers and fellow counselors, finding genuine camaraderie, and his eyes sparkled with delight whenever he talked about his camp experiences.

Working at the MDA camp provided him with the opportunity to make a positive impact on others' lives, and he found a sense of self-worth and pride in meaningful work. It brought us immense joy to witness his dedication to caring for others, and his unselfish, loving commitment to the MDA camp fills us with pride to this day.

However, despite the overall positive nature of his camp experience, it did not yield the intended outcome regarding his substance use. Randy Michael continued to use marijuana, and his behavior became more dangerous and damaging to himself and our family. Today I know that our hopes for breaking Randy Michael's compulsive like marijuana habit and the methods we pursued were somewhat idealistic. We were simply unaware of the insidious power of drug addiction, further compounded by marijuana's current potency and its addictive nature.[10]

---

10 B. J. Arterberry, H. Treloar Padovano, K. T. Foster, R. A. Zucker RA, and B. M. Hicks, "Higher Average Potency across the United States Is Associated with Progression to First Cannabis Use Disorder Symptom," *Drug and Alcohol Dependence* 195 (2019): 186–92, https://doi:10.1016/j.drugalcdep.2018.11.012

CHAPTER 4

TURBULENT LOVE

High School Battles

Although Randy Michael's experience at the MDA camp was positive, the remainder of the summer before his junior year of high school was turbulent. More than once, we discovered he had sneaked out of the house, often joining peers who made questionable choices.

Near the end of the summer, Randy Michael was sleeping over at a friend's home when his friend's parents stumbled upon a backpack containing weed. The boys concocted a clever tale to shield their host, who owned the backpack, asserting it belonged to a student from a different school who was also at the party.

After this incident, we decided Randy Michael would not attend any more sleepovers—especially because we learned that sleepovers served as a way for the kids to avoid returning home while under the influence of substances like alcohol or marijuana. Randy Michael was angry with us, but we were increasingly aware of his frequent substance use, and our growing concern for his well-being overshadowed our concern about his frustration.

In late September 2016, shortly after Randy Michael began his junior year of high school, another troubling incident occurred. I was away visiting Brooke at college, and my husband, Randy, was home with our other three children. Around midnight, Randy Michael returned home from a Saturday evening out with friends. He bid his father goodnight and headed to his bedroom. At 4 a.m., Randy's phone rang.

"Hello, Mr. Bacchus? This is the Washington County sheriff; we have your son and a couple of his friends. We found them in a park with a significant amount of marijuana in their possession. Both edibles and smokable."

When Randy arrived to pick up our son, he noticed the other parents, then heard the "cool mom" say, "Don't be too harsh on them. They're just kids."

Even though Randy Michael claimed sole ownership of the drugs, we suspect he was choosing to take responsibility because he didn't want any of his friends to get into more trouble; he was never one to throw others under the bus.

Randy Michael could have been charged with a felony due to the quantity of edibles he possessed. However, because it was his first offense and because he behaved like a polite and respectful young man, he was charged only with a misdemeanor.

Randy Michael had been in counseling since his sophomore year of high school, and we again sought professional assistance from his therapist as our frustration and worry grew over his behavior. Both my husband and I attended his therapy sessions monthly, expressing to the therapist our concerns about his choices. We maintained consequences for Randy Michael's actions and attempted to help him understand our perspective, expressing our genuine worry and care for his well-being.

Regrettably, much of this seemed to fall on deaf ears. Perhaps it was just the typical defiance of a sixteen-year-old, or maybe Randy Michael was not entirely forthcoming with the therapist. He just seemed to grow angrier. When he would look at me, his eyes were blank, cold, and empty. It seemed as if our son was slowly disappearing. He became increasingly distant, defiant, anxious, and combative—steadfastly maintaining that marijuana was harmless and even beneficial for him. We were unaware at the time how such beliefs are widespread among marijuana users and throughout the industry that profits off addiction.

> ## *You Need to Know*
>
> As noted above, marijuana/cannabis use during adolescence poses a higher risk for the user to develop a cannabis use disorder. Also, adolescent onset of use is associated with other negative consequences, including addiction, anxiety, depression, restlessness, irritability, and psychosis that is largely attributed to THC.[11]
>
> Research shows that how adolescents and young adults perceive cannabis can be a major driver of whether and how they use it. Regular users typically view the risks of cannabis as low, and as more and more young people consume it in various forms, fewer of them view it as posing any significant danger.[12]

In one family session, I shared that Randy Michael had admitted to driving his sisters to school while high, and I was shocked and disturbed by the therapist's response.

---

11 Marie-Eve Di Raddo et al., "Δ9-Tetrahydrocannabinol Does Not Upregulate an Aversive Dopamine Receptor Mechanism in Adolescent Brain Unlike in Adults," *Current Research in Neurobiology* 5 (September 2023), https://doi.org/10.1016/j.crneur.2023.100107.

12 Nhung Nguyen et al., "Adolescents' and Young Adults' Perceptions of Risks and Benefits Differ by Type of Cannabis Products," *Addictive Behaviors* 131 (2022), https://doi.org/10.1016/j.addbeh.2022.107336.

"Driving high isn't that bad," he told us. "Most people just drive slower."

I was infuriated by this response. I felt unsupported. Now I know his statement disregarded the growing evidence of the dangers of driving under the influence of marijuana. These dangers are becoming especially apparent in states like Colorado, where marijuana legalization occurred in 2013.

> ### *You Need to Know*
>
> Statistics from the Rocky Mountain High Intensity Drug Trafficking Area (HIDTA) Investigative Support Center in 2021 revealed a 138 percent increase in traffic deaths involving drivers who tested positive for marijuana since legalization. In addition, there has been a 29 percent surge in overall traffic fatalities.[13] A review of the research literature on driving safety and marijuana use concluded that after inhaling THC, users should wait at least five hours before operating a motor vehicle.[14]

Desperate to Control the Chaos

By early in his junior year of high school, at the tender age of sixteen, Randy Michael had drained all our energy reserves, and our daughters were constantly exposed to our ongoing conflicts over his

---

13 "2021 Marijuana Report—The Legalization of Marijuana in Colorado: The Impact (vol. 8)," Rocky Mountain HIDTA, September 2021, https://www.rmhidta.org/publications?pgid=khxvk038-6a0e2823-f0e2-4f73-b236-34dfc9e4952d.

14 Danielle McCartney, Thomas R. Arkell, Christopher Irwin, and Iain S. McGregor, "Determining the Magnitude and Duration of Acute Δ9-Tetrahydrocannabinol (Δ9-THC)-Induced Driving and Cognitive Impairment: A Systematic and Meta-analytic Review," *Neuroscience & Biobehavioral Reviews* (January 2021), https://doi.org/10.1016/j.neubiorev.2021.01.003.

disrespect and aggressive behavior. Our household had spiraled into complete chaos. Following the possession incident in September, we carefully navigated the insurance system to have Randy Michael evaluated at a local clinic that specializes in mental health and addiction. His diagnosis of a cannabis use disorder (CUD) qualified him for admission to an inpatient treatment center.

Looking back, I realize we were in denial and having difficulty accepting how serious our son's situation had become. Despite Randy Michael's diagnosis and the chaos we were living in, we hesitated to make the next move, questioning whether he genuinely required inpatient treatment at that time. If we sent him to treatment, it meant that we were admitting that our son had a serious addiction. We feared the label and stigma of being considered "an addict" and we wanted to protect him. We also felt responsible for our son's behavior and ashamed to admit how bad it had become.

However, an evening in October 2016 opened our eyes to the true problem—the straw that broke the camel's back. Up until this point, we had never seen or experienced firsthand the evidence of Randy Michael using marijuana in our presence or our home. He had always been caught after the fact, and never by us.

There was no more denying our son had a problem. When we returned home that evening from an event, we entered our house through the back door and discovered that the entire house reeked! "Oh my gosh, a skunk must have gotten inside," I told my husband, Randy.

As I stood in our back entryway, reality hit me like a brick wall. I quickly realized there had been no skunk in the house. I was smelling the pungent odor of weed. Heat surged from my toes to my face, and my heart was pounding as I ran downstairs to Randy Michael's bedroom.

Rap music was blaring. I flung open his bathroom door, and a cloud of steam carried the skunkiest aroma into the house. Randy Michael, high as a kite, was enjoying his shower. He had fashioned an "apple pipe"—a homemade smoking device—from an apple core and a toilet paper roll. (Need a tutorial? Multiple videos on YouTube demonstrate how to craft such devices from everyday items.)

He apparently thought he would have time to hide any evidence before we returned. But our home's front doors had been removed for refinishing, so when he opened his window to smoke, a backdraft carried the pungent and thick aroma of highly potent marijuana through our entire house.

We were a mix of fury, concern, frustration, sadness, and worry, realizing this was a breaking point. In an act of desperation and naivety, seeking any sort of help, we rushed Randy Michael to the local hospital for detox. However, since it was "just weed," they would not keep him. In the belly of the hospital, we met with a social worker who did not understand the chaos Randy Michael brought to our house. She gave us no resources or direction, and we returned home more frustrated than ever, and now with an unnecessary emergency department bill from a futile visit.

Living with Randy Michael had become unbearable. He was argumentative and defiant, and we were constantly walking on eggshells in his presence. The next weekend Randy Michael began threatening me, harassing me, spitting at me, cursing at me, and calling me names, and he became physically aggressive against his dad; it was terrifying. Exhausted and fearful, we called 911. We had no idea that "just weed" could provoke such behavior, particularly in adolescents diagnosed with a cannabis use disorder.[15]

---

[15] Will Lawn et al., "The CannTeen Study: Cannabis Use Disorder, Depression, Anxiety, and Psychotic-Like Symptoms in Adolescent and Adult Cannabis Users and Age-Matched Controls," *Journal of Psychopharmacology* 36, no. 12 (2022): 1350–61, https://doi.org/10.1177/02698811221108956.

County police officers arrived and helped calm the situation. They reaffirmed our parental right to establish rules and enforce consequences for Randy Michael's behavior.

> ### You Need to Know
>
> Adolescent cannabis users have a greater propensity compared to adult users to experience psychotic-like symptoms and poorer mental health in the presence of a cannabis use disorder.[16]

After that incident, we decided to send Randy Michael to a wilderness camp in Utah. Our decision was based in part on the advice of a fellow parent facing a similar challenge, an interventionist who is also a family friend, and the therapist I was seeing at the time. The hope was that the outdoor experience, coupled with education, would foster resilience, independence, and emotional growth, to help him cope and process his emotions, which still included grief over the loss of his friend Aaron.

We did not want to resort to the drastic measures used by some camps and parents called "gooning"—a process where a couple of men forcibly take a defiant teen away in the dead of night to treatment or a wilderness camp. Instead, we engaged in open discussions about the camp we wanted Randy Michael to attend. Eventually, after many, many hours of discussion, he agreed to go. Reluctant, sad, and broken, Randy Michael departed for Utah with his dad by his side in October 2016.

We were out of energy and ideas, but we knew Randy Michael needed professional help. Randy returned exhausted from drop-

---

16 C. J. Hammond et al., "Cannabis Use among U.S. Adolescents in the Era of Marijuana Legalization: A Review of Changing Use Patterns, Comorbidity, and Health Correlates," *International Review of Psychiatry* 32, no. 3 (2020): 221–34, https://doi.org/10.1080/09540261.2020.1713056.

ping Randy Michael off in Utah, having cried the entire flight home. Sending Randy Michael away was an agonizing but crucial decision; our household needed respite. Although we had high hopes for the camp, our lives would only grow more complicated from that point onward.

> ### You Need to Know
>
> Some educational consultants specialize in finding the right treatment and school for youth suffering from addiction. Although it comes at a cost, it is often worth the investment to find the place that will give a loved one the best chance of a successful and sustained recovery. Consider using an educational consultant for the likelihood of greater success.

No Miracles in the Wilderness

Randy Michael spent nine grueling weeks in Utah. He slept in a tent on a thin mat, cooked his food, and used an outdoor latrine or a bag to be disposed of later. Everything he owned, he carried in a backpack on his shoulders. He left home weighing around two hundred pounds and returned about thirty pounds lighter, thin as a rail.

The young male campers lived on the trails, taking classes, and engaging in group and individual therapy sessions. We had weekly family therapy with Randy Michael via the phone, exchanged letters, and did our therapy homework assignments, which consisted of reading assigned books and setting expectations. Randy and I made a one-weekend visit with our son, where we participated in rock climbing excursions, family therapy sessions, and shared meals. But we left with heavy hearts. Randy Michael appeared alarmingly thin, and he made it clear that he still believed marijuana was harmless and there was no need for him to stop using it.

Filled with the uncertainty about Randy Michael transitioning home soon and worried because his attitude had not changed, this time I was the one to cry all the way home on the flight from Utah. The wilderness camp leaders suggested we enroll Randy Michael in a therapeutic boarding school. The concept sounded promising, but like many families, we could not afford the seven-thousand-dollar monthly tab.

You Need to Know

There are such things as "sober" high schools and colleges, although they are not as prevalent as they should be. For example, Minnesota used to have twenty-six sober high schools. As of 2024, we have six schools that are active members of the Association of Recovery Schools. Sober high schools have been proven to increase student sobriety and probability of high school graduation.[17] Had I known about that option, I would have sent Randy Michael to a sober school in our neighboring school district.

During Randy Michael's stay at the wilderness camp, he underwent his fourth comprehensive psychological evaluation. The diagnoses mirrored earlier assessments, highlighting ADHD, a processing disorder, and low executive functioning skills. However, this time he was also diagnosed with oppositional defiant disorder (only with his parents), anxiety, and depression. Once again, Randy Michael displayed exceptional verbal fluency, writing skills, and memorization abilities. While these findings were consistent with previous evaluations, the addition of oppositional defiant disorder, anxiety, and depression shed light on

---

17 D. L. Weimer et al., "Net Benefits of Recovery High Schools: Higher Cost but Increased Sobriety and Educational Attainment," *Journal of Mental Health Policy and Economics* 22, no. 3 (2019): 109–20, https://pubmed.ncbi.nlm.nih.gov/31811754/.

the potential impact of marijuana use on his adolescent mental health—an unfortunate realization that eluded us at the time.[18]

> **You Need to Know**
>
> Numerous research studies show that regular and consistent use of cannabis is associated with poorer educational outcomes and an increased level of depressive symptoms.[19] Depressive symptoms and disruptive behavior disorders often accompany cannabis use disorders, especially in individuals with ADHD, conduct disorder, or oppositional defiant disorder.
>
> A child who struggles with ADHD has a higher likelihood of also struggling with cannabis use or a cannabis use disorder. Parents who have a child with ADHD need to understand this and how it can impact their child and their future.[20]

A Rocky Return

After nine weeks of wilderness therapy, we decided Randy Michael should return home right before Christmas. He was eager to go back to his former high school, but we were concerned about his circle of friends there. We enrolled him in our local public high school.

---

18 M. C. Morse, K. Benson, and K. Flory, "Disruptive Behavior Disorders and Marijuana Use: The Role of Depressive Symptoms," *Substance Abuse: Research and Treatment*, August 28, 2016, https://doi.org/10.4137/SART.S31432.

19 Ileana Pacheco-Colón et al., "Effects of Adolescent Cannabis Use on Motivation and Depression: A Systematic Review," *Current Addiction Reports* 6, no. 4 (2019): 532–46, https://doi.org/10.1007/s40429-019-00274-y.

20 Trine Tollerup Nielsen, Jinjie Duan, Daniel F. Levey, G. Bragi Walters, Emma C. Johnson, Thorgeir Thorgeirsson, Thomas Werge, et al., "Shared Genetics of ADHD, Cannabis Use Disorder and Cannabis Use and Prediction of Cannabis Use Disorder in ADHD," *Nature Mental Health* (July 2024), 1–13, https://doi.org/10.1038/s44220-024-00277-3.

With the help of a camp therapist, we had established clear boundaries and created a family contract before Randy Michael returned home. Random drug tests were part of the arrangement to ensure compliance so that he could earn back privileges. To be allowed to drive again, Randy Michael would have to maintain a drug-free status with clean test results. We also made the difficult decision to withhold his phone while he was at school, knowing it could be a tool to access marijuana. In our conversations, we made it clear to Randy Michael that if he was determined to use marijuana, he would have to live elsewhere.

To say Randy Michael was unhappy at home would be an understatement. We knew it wouldn't be easy for him to adjust to a new school in his junior year—a challenge even in the best of circumstances. Despite having connections with some kids at school from playing sports and from grade school, he told me it was "cliquey." He was so unhappy.

Eventually, his struggles led him back to old habits, and he was caught vaping in the bathroom, breaching our zero-tolerance contract. We presented him with two choices: He could agree not to smoke or move out. It may sound stern, but he had been requesting legal emancipation from our family for more than a year. So, in the spring of his junior year, our seventeen-year-old son moved out of our home.

Randy Michael left on a rainy spring evening in 2017, carrying his bag and a mix of sadness and frustration. We were deeply concerned for him but determined to let him make his choice. I provided him with a list of teen shelters in our area complete with addresses and phone numbers.

Before he left, I offered up a prayer to the Virgin Mary, seeking her guidance and care for Randy Michael. It seemed she did watch over him. Our neighbor's son picked him up that evening, and he ended up staying just three doors away on the opposite side of the street. We learned about his whereabouts through the neighborhood grapevine.

It took three weeks before those neighbors reached out to us to let us know that Randy Michael was in their home. Their silence frustrated me. I knew that if one of my children brought home a friend, I would immediately contact the parents to get a better understanding of the full situation and let them know that their child was safe. While I appreciated the neighbors' willingness to support our son, I wished they would have communicated with us so that they could have fully comprehended our family situation.

Despite Randy Michael living elsewhere, we maintained contact through texts. He continued to argue that pot was good for him. He said it was calming, helped him to focus and sleep, and made him more creative. We said when he was prepared to stop using and ready to follow our rules, he could come home. After about two months and with the help of a therapist, Randy Michael agreed not to use and returned home for the summer.

While he was home that summer, Randy Michael adhered to our house rules, worked, and demonstrated forward-thinking about his future.

Planning for the Future

The spring semester of junior year is critical for high schoolers looking to attend college for so many reasons, including scheduling standardized tests and college visits. Randy Michael had ambitious dreams of attending the University of Colorado in Boulder—a location where he could indulge his love for skiing and the mountains. He had visited as a sophomore and was determined to go there. Despite all the turmoil during his high school years, Randy Michael astounded us by scoring a remarkable 28 on his ACT.

He wasn't living at home when he took his test, and his joy was infectious when he called to tell us his score. We were elated by his score but disheartened when he claimed he had done so well because he had used marijuana the night before the test.

To assist our family with Randy Michael's return home that summer, we pursued the help of a therapist. Unfortunately, this therapist refused to believe that his marijuana use was a real problem. In front of Randy Michael and Sabrina, she falsely claimed that 75 percent of kids use marijuana. I firmly disagreed with her and emphasized that marijuana use was not acceptable in our home or for our son—regardless of her statistics. It was so unsettling to me that she had undermined our position right in front of our children, despite being fully aware of our family's struggle. It left me feeling minimized, defeated, and frustrated.

You Need to Know

When seeking help from a professional therapist or counselor, thoroughly vet them to ensure their advice will align with your family's values and needs. Ask about their knowledge of recent research on drug use and the issues and problems relevant to your child. Look for a licensed professional who specializes in drug and alcohol counseling if you are dealing with a substance-use matter.

Also, be ready to dispel beliefs that use is very common among youth. According to the 2022 *Monitoring the Future* survey, roughly 30.7 percent of high school seniors reported using cannabis/hashish in the past twelve months. That means 69.3 percent of seniors have not.[21] That is a far cry from 75 percent of kids using.

---

21 National Institute on Drug Abuse, "What Is the Scope of Cannabis (Marijuana) Use in the United States?," December 2023, https://nida.nih.gov/publications/research-reports/marijuana/what-scope-marijuana-use-in-united-states.

Despite my lack of faith in this therapist, she did play a role in convincing Randy Michael to agree not to smoke and to consider attending a boarding school for his senior year. We believed that attending a boarding school might prepare him for college while also granting him the independence he had wanted for nearly two years. We explored various options and eventually settled on a Christian-based inner-city school on Chicago's West Side, valuing its diversity, alignment with our beliefs, and affordability.

CHAPTER 5

TOUGH LOVE

Senior Year

As we prepared to send Randy Michael to boarding school for his senior year of high school, we met with the school's founder and the two "house fathers," who oversaw the boarding house where Randy Michael lived and who were fully aware of Randy Michael's struggles. I had mixed emotions when we dropped him off, hopeful that the school would offer him a new start, yet fearful for his well-being because he was living far away for the first time on the West Side of Chicago and had a history of marijuana use.

We visited Randy Michael at the boarding house a few different times in the fall, usually as we passed through Chicago on our way to visit Brooke, who was a junior at Notre Dame in South Bend, Indiana. Our visits were not always encouraging. At times, he resisted our presence, objecting even to simple requests like using the bathroom in his boardinghouse. The house seemed disorderly and was dirty. The two teachers overseeing the young men living there didn't hold any protective or parental role—not what I had expected house fathers to be.

Later we realized there was a significant lack of supervision at the house, which was a serious concern, especially for our son. We also realized he had not wanted us to enter the house because he wanted to conceal signs of his marijuana use. We deeply regret sending him to that school. At the time we believed it was the right choice, but that is one of many decisions I would now make differently.

Randy Michael had landed a job at a local hot dog shop while living in Chicago. He was happy to be making money and gaining work experience. But he was struggling at school, which he told us was because he did not have an individualized education program (IEP). Unfortunately, denial can cloud perception profoundly, and we naively missed the signs that our son was once again using marijuana regularly, even though we knew that he was attending school and living with peers who were entangled in gang culture.

Randy Michael often compassionately shared stories about his classmates' challenging home lives—highlighting that sports or academics were their only escape routes from a tough life on Chicago's West Side. He used to tell me, "Mom, you have no idea what their lives are like." And he was right: I truly did not. Ultimately, I did not know what his life was like either.

Throughout the semester, Randy Michael called home frequently. He complained of stomach issues and took numerous sick days. I would suggest that he try a gluten-free diet, and I suspected his upset stomach might have been caused by drinking too much. He also told me that he spent extended periods in the steam shower in the house and how much he loved it.

Later, I learned about a condition called cannabis hyperemesis syndrome that can cause persistent nausea and vomiting.[22] It is

---

22 Jonathan A. Galli et al., "Cannabinoid Hyperemesis Syndrome," *Current Drug Abuse Reviews* 4, no. 4 (2011): 241–49, https://doi.org/10.2174/18744737111040 40241.

relieved only by hot showers or by smoking more marijuana.[23] I am pretty certain Randy Michael's use was causing him to feel nauseated and that the steam shower probably helped relieve symptoms.

Unexpected Expulsion

In the third week of December 2017, I received an alarming call from Randy Michael's school: he was being expelled and needed to take his finals and leave the premises within twenty-four hours! School leaders claimed Randy Michael had been playing pranks in the boarding house despite warnings to stop. For Randy Michael, known to procrastinate but pull through with decent grades on finals, this sudden move left him utterly frustrated, and he feared—with good reason—that this expulsion would mar his college prospects.

With no time to study, he ended up failing all his finals. As a result of his expulsion, his marijuana use, and his failure, he was deeply anxious, angry, and struggling upon returning home.

Randy Michael believed it was "unfair" that he had been asked to leave school with no notice, and we were also intensely frustrated with the school's lack of communication. Had we been aware of his disruptive behavior at the boarding house, we would have implemented consequences, such as disabling his cell phone. Unfortunately, the school never reached out to us, even though we had attended in-person conferences in the fall. At that time, no teacher and neither house father mentioned any issues beyond his below-average grades, a somewhat common occurrence for Randy Michael, who would often slack off for months and then

---

23 C. J. Sorensen et al., "Cannabinoid Hyperemesis Syndrome: Diagnosis, Pathophysiology, and Treatment—A Systematic Review," *Journal of Medical Toxicology* 13 (2017): 71–87, https://doi.org/10.1007/s13181-016-0595-z.

pull his grades up by working very hard at the end of the semester. He had managed to maintain a B average throughout high school following this pattern.

We did not know how frequently he was using drugs that fall, which likely contributed significantly to his unacceptable behavior and declining grades. We did not know it at the time because like most people suffering from addiction, Randy Michael had not been honest with us about his substance use.

We empathized with Randy Michael even though we tried to make him comprehend the repercussions of his actions. We always tried to teach our children that wise choices typically yield positive outcomes, while poor choices often lead to bad ones. Unfortunately, this message didn't seem to resonate with Randy Michael. Maybe he just couldn't see it because he sincerely believed that marijuana was good—and immediately after using it, it made him feel high and euphoric. However, his cannabis use disorder prevented him from seeing the negatives it brought into his life.

You Need to Know

Cannabis use can cause an average of an eight-point drop in IQ if use begins during adolescence and continues into adulthood, according to longitudinal studies.[24], [25]

Although I knew he was struggling, I didn't realize the extent of his unhappiness or drug use when he was in Chicago until

---

24 Emmet Power et al., "Intelligence Quotient Decline following Frequent or Dependent Cannabis Use in Youth: A Systematic Review and Meta-analysis of Longitudinal Studies," *Psychological Medicine* 51, no. 2 (2021): 194–200, https://doi.org/10.1017/S0033291720005036.

25 R. S. Sultan et al., "Nondisordered Cannabis Use among US Adolescents," *JAMA Network Open* 6, no. 5 (2023), https://doi.org/10.1001/jamanetworkopen.2023.11294.

I read through Randy Michael's letters and journals after his death. Here is an excerpt from a letter he wrote to a girl from high school whom he had spent time with the previous summer.

January 2019

I am sorry for harassing you after all the times you hung out with me that summer. I honestly thought you were beautiful and struggled with myself at the time. When I sent you that first message that made you block me, I was on drugs and was listening to shitty advice friends in Chicago had given me. I just wanted to impress you and thought of you as a very beautiful and cool girl, and seeing you pull away crushed me because I let it. I also was never confident around you, so it probably was just a distorted dream of you and me having something at some point. I hope you go on to live a fruitful life. Thanks for being nice to me that summer. You were the only light in my life at the time. I wouldn't forgive myself either.

In that excerpt, a lot is happening. He admits to using, clearly carrying shame for past words and actions, while also deeply admiring this girl and seeking her approval. In hindsight, I think Randy Michael began this quest for acceptance in ninth grade; unfortunately, weed provided a very temporary solution to find the acceptance he craved.

Anger and Aggression

Now eighteen, Randy Michael's months in the boardinghouse had given him a certain level of freedom from supervision. That freedom had allowed for easy access to drugs, and his use had spiraled. At home under watchful eyes, he had less access to substances, his main coping strategy, and his struggles with his behavior and his moods were intensifying.

As the second semester of his senior year approached, tensions were high, particularly as we discussed plans for future schooling. Randy Michael wanted to return to his former private high school, yet we were apprehensive to send him there, knowing many of his peers were still engaging in risky behavior. It was clear to both Randy and me that reintegrating our son into that environment wouldn't be in his best interest. We offered options, including the local public school, alternative learning centers, or online schooling. Randy Michael wanted nothing to do with any of those. We even suggested that he get his GED. Honestly, at this point, we just wanted him to get a high school degree.

On Christmas Day in 2017, I hosted a festive gathering for twenty-three members of our family—ten adults and thirteen kids and teens. Every corner of the house was filled as we bustled around preparing food and entertaining our guests. Somehow, amid all the activity, no one realized that Randy Michael had been drinking throughout the day. In our family, celebrations do not revolve around alcohol, so no one was on the lookout for this kind of excess.

After enjoying a big dinner, exchanging presents, and indulging in dessert, we gathered downstairs to watch movies, only to discover Randy Michael was already in bed. It struck me as odd, but I knew he was unhappy, so I simply let him sleep.

A few days later, while Randy Michael was at work at Fleet Farm General Store, one of his sisters suggested that we clean out his room and look underneath his mattress. When we lifted it, we discovered several empty beer and wine bottles—clearly Randy Michael had been drinking alone, likely on multiple occasions. Eventually, he admitted that he fell ill on Christmas Day after consuming an old bottle of wine—one I had kept for display purposes only.

I hoped Randy Michael had learned that drinking alone and taking liquor from us were not good ideas. But his behavior worried me and made me very sad. What was happening to our son?

In January 2018, he resumed trying to convince us that marijuana was medicinal and good for him. He insisted it was a lifesaver, brought him happiness, and was harmless due to its natural origin. But his attempts at persuasion were filled with aggression, verbal abuse, and anger. One day, I was at the grocery store when he began bombarding me with text messages.

"Will you allow me to smoke weed at home? I need an answer by 5 p.m., or I will kill myself."

He persisted with relentless messages, demanding a reply. When I refused, he would text "Mom, Mom, Mom" at least fifty times in succession. Then he would resort to further threats and attempts to coerce us into permitting drug use in our home.

One evening that month, a noticeably agitated Randy Michael again insisted on arguing about marijuana, vehemently trying to justify the benefits of smoking. When we refused to permit him to use in our home, he stormed out of the house in a fit of rage. On the second consecutive night, as he exited through the front doors with a belt in his hand, dropping his cell phone on the entryway rug, and walking out the front door he exclaimed, "If you won't let me smoke marijuana, then I am going to kill myself!"

We felt scared, worried, overwhelmed, frustrated, and upset. None of this should have been happening. My heart was racing; all three of our daughters were sobbing.

You Need to Know

Several studies point to an increase in suicidal ideation for adolescents using high-potency cannabis.[26] A notable example is Colorado. Since the legalization of marijuana, the suicide rate across all age groups has risen significantly, increasing over 30 percent between 2013 and 2022. During that same period, suicides involving marijuana have increased more than 2.4 times. In 2021, marijuana was the most frequently detected substance in the systems of young people aged twenty-four and under from Colorado who committed suicide. Marijuana was present in 34.9 percent of suicides among individuals aged ten to twenty-four, compared to alcohol, which was found in 33.1 percent of cases within that age group.[27]

Frightened, we urgently contacted the local police to help find our son. It was the second time we had called on them that month to help locate him. The first night, the girls had successfully located their brother and brought him home. However, this night, the police found Randy Michael at a nearby gas station and intervened, taking him to the hospital where he was admitted to the psychiatric ward and placed under a mandatory three-day hold for evaluation and care.

Navigating in the Dark

We hated to see him in the psych ward, and Randy Michael pleaded with us to bring him home before his three days were

---

26 Kristen Schmidt et al., "A Systematic Review: Adolescent Cannabis Use and Suicide," *Addictive Disorders & Their Treatment* 19, no. 3 (September 2020): 146–51, https://doi.org/10.1097/ADT.0000000000000196.

27 Colorado Department of Health and Environment, "Workbook: COVDRS Suicide Dashboard All Years Excludes Race," 2021, https://cohealthviz.dphe.state.co.us/t/HealthInformaticsPublic/views/COVDRSSuicideDashboardAllYearsExcludesRace/Story1?%3Aembed=y&%3Aiid=1&%3AisGuestRedirectFromVizportal=y.

up. But our family was at a total loss, facing a crisis without a clue how to navigate it. Randy Michael's disruptive behavior at home was affecting our girls, who saw him berating us, becoming aggressive, and threatening his own life. They were afraid of him and afraid for him.

It was clear that he valued marijuana more than his own life or his relationship with others. He staunchly insisted marijuana was medicinal for him and suggested that we would rather see him dead than allow him to smoke. His addicted mindset was utterly irrational.

While Randy Michael was hospitalized, we consulted with the on-staff psychiatrist, who suggested that he could be on the autism spectrum. This was the first time a professional had raised such a possibility. I struggled with that idea then and now—especially considering Randy Michael's prior psychological assessments and her awareness of his history of cannabis use. His cannabis consumption had resulted in manifestations of depression, anxiety, defiance, aggression, and suicidal ideation—we didn't even have the slightest concern about autism.

Although Randy Michael's marijuana usage was disclosed to all medical professionals and therapists he interacted with, none attributed his difficult behavior to substance abuse. This hospital stay marked the onset of what we believe was a series of misdiagnoses that Randy Michael encountered while grappling with his addiction.

Due to the turmoil Randy Michael had caused at home, we made the difficult decision that he couldn't return to live with us when he was discharged from the hospital after his three-day hold. Randy Michael was eighteen years old, which complicated matters significantly. In the eyes of the state, he was considered an adult. He was not obligated to accept any treatment, nor was he required to share his medical records with us or let us communicate with his care providers. Thankfully, he had granted us access to his medical records and allowed us to talk with his doctors.

> ### *You Need to Know*
>
> Once your loved one turns eighteen, they have the legal right to refuse treatment unless they choose to seek help voluntarily. Additionally, they are not required to grant you access to their medical information or communicate with their healthcare providers.
>
> If you want to stay informed about their care and condition, it's crucial to have a medical release of information signed. This document will allow professionals to share important details with you, ensuring you're kept in the loop.

Overwhelmed, I was hoping the hospital would assign him a social worker, but they did not. No one on the care team gave Randy Michael or us any guidance or resources for next steps after he left the hospital.

We felt lost. Thankfully, a relative offered to take him in under the condition that he abstain from using, enroll in school, attend psychiatric sessions, and undergo therapy.

We attempted to seek treatment for Randy Michael at a nearby psychiatry clinic specializing in aiding youth dealing with mental health and substance abuse issues. They diagnosed Randy Michael with dysthymia, a mild but long-lasting form of depression, and prescribed medication. However, Randy Michael refused to disclose the medication's name to me and discontinued it after just one night, citing disturbing dreams as a side effect. Randy Michael was bright and resourceful, and I am guessing he researched the medication's side effects and chose to stop it based on what he read.

I wish that before he took his first hit at 15, he had researched the scientific studies highlighting the negative effects of high-potency marijuana on the developing adolescent brain. Had he known the truth about today's highly potent marijuana, not just the industry propaganda, maybe then, he would never have started using it.

> ## *You Need to Know*
>
> Adolescents with a cannabis use disorder are at an elevated risk of suffering from a decrease in executive functioning, impaired cognitive functioning, and deficits in decision-making because cannabis use interferes with the functional connectivity in the thinking part of the brain—the prefrontal cortex. The prefrontal cortex, the final region of the brain to complete neurological development during youth, primarily houses the executive functioning skills necessary to negotiate the teenage years and become a successful adult. These skills include time management, decision-making, impulsivity, planning, attention, organization, perseverance, working memory, and flexibility.[28] Avoiding cannabis use while the brain is developing can help adolescents become successful adults.

After two days of school and therapy sessions at the clinic, Randy Michael refused to continue taking classes. He vehemently disliked the environment, claiming the other kids there were more troubled or odd than he was. He said he felt an inability to connect with anyone. We insisted he continue therapy and see the psychiatrist.

---

28 Jazmin Camchong et al., "Adverse Effects of Cannabis on Adolescent Brain Development: A Longitudinal Study," *Cerebral Cortex* 27, no. 3 (March 2017): 1922–30, https://doi.org/10.1093/cercor/bhw015.

This psychiatrist, unlike other doctors, implemented routine drug testing—a significant relief for us, as previous doctors, particularly family physicians, had disregarded our requests for these tests.

> ## *You Need to Know*
>
> I wish we had started randomly drug-testing Randy Michael when he was in seventh grade. That way he could have told his friends he could not use drugs. If you're thinking about going this route, you should know that kids can purchase fake urine online or add a drop of bleach to a urine test to make it inconclusive.
>
> Testing ordered by a doctor and done at the doctor's office leaves less room for cheating. Yet testing for active THC in urine does not necessarily provide an accurate picture of current use versus prior use. Keep in mind the lingering presence of THC in urine: a positive test could mean there is a recent drug-free period, but use occurred weeks earlier.

With clean drug tests at the psychiatry office, Randy Michael started taking Concerta again for his ADHD and eventually transitioned to an online schooling program. The semester was incredibly challenging because he tended to procrastinate, and we learned that he had started using marijuana once again. We were concerned he would not graduate. Our rocky road continued.

Because Randy Michael had lost his driving privileges due to his marijuana use, we regularly drove him to his appointments and to and from work. During each ride, he begged us to move back home. Eventually, we established clear conditions for his return: he must abstain from smoking, continue to see his therapist and a psychiatrist, adhere to the household rules, maintain employment, and complete his high school education online. He finally agreed to these terms, and we welcomed him back into our house.

Although he had fallen behind in his online classes, Randy Michael worked hard to catch up so he could graduate, and he began making plans for life after high school. Although we tried to convince him to stay closer to home, he desperately wanted to attend the University of Colorado–Boulder. When he was accepted there, he declared his intentions to join a fraternity and made it clear that he "wanted to party and partying is what college is all about."

Given his strong determination and his desire to party, we proposed that Randy Michael take a gap year and establish residency in Colorado. We explained that once he demonstrated responsibility and settled into his new environment, we would consider assisting him with his schooling. He eventually agreed to take a gap year while living in Colorado and established his residency.

Between April and August 12, 2018, Randy Michael graduated high school online, bought a car from us and insured it, secured an apartment, landed a job as a bank teller in Boulder, and packed up his belongings for a move. We made it clear that he would be responsible for rent and all his living expenses. Together, he and I created a budget based on his expected income.

The only thing we provided for was his cell phone. We wanted to ensure that he would have less money to spend on weed and that we would not be enabling his habit.

You Need to Know

The second-biggest holiday in cannabis culture is 710 Day, or 7/10, which falls on July 10 each year. Celebrated for the past decade, the date is derived from the word "OIL" when turned upside down and spelled backward: 710. On this day, enthusiasts consume cannabis oils, dabs, or concentrates at 7:10 a.m. or 7:10 p.m. or both. It's similar to 420 Day, but specifically celebrates the use of highly potent dab products.

CHAPTER 6

LOVE OF FREEDOM

Moving to Colorado

We threw Randy Michael a going-away party with close family and friends. I treasure photos from that evening because many were lasts. On August 12, 2018, Randy Michael and his dad departed for Boulder. In photos from that day, my concern and mixed emotions about my son's move are evident in my puffy face and worried expressions.

As they pulled out of the driveway, tears filled my eyes and knots turned in the pit of my stomach. I was so worried for Randy Michael's well-being and safety. Although living his dream, my heart and head were concerned.

Once in Boulder, Randy Michael settled into his new life, started his job, and maintained occasional contact with us. From the very beginning of his time in Colorado, he voiced frustration about missing out on freshman events at the University of Colorado and how difficult it was to connect with his peers because he wasn't in class like a "normal" freshman. Gradually, his communication with us dwindled, and I sensed he'd made new friends and was getting more and more involved in social and party activities.

When he did talk with us, he would complain about stomach issues—aches, nausea, and diarrhea. Initially, I considered the possibility of food sensitivity, but now I suspect his fast-paced lifestyle and marijuana use might have contributed to his stomach problems, especially as I have learned more about cannabis hyperemesis syndrome, which causes intestinal issues in longtime marijuana users.[29]

You Need to Know

Another name for cannabis hyperemesis syndrome (CHS) is "scrommiting." This phrase was coined by Dr. Rohnet Lev, an Emergency Department doctor in San Diego when she saw multiple patients vomiting and screaming because of extreme abdominal pain. Screaming + vomiting = scrommiting.

Regular cannabis users may experience this syndrome as cyclical bouts of nausea, vomiting, and abdominal pain that can lead to dehydration.[30] Immediate relief can be found in hot showers—or by using more cannabis. Permanent relief can come from the cessation of cannabis use.

Since the legalization of cannabis in Colorado, a notable increase in CHS cases has been recorded, with doctors witnessing a surge in Emergency Department visits due to this condition. Some individuals have even lost their lives to it.[31]

---

29 J. E. Fleming and S. Lockwood, "Cannabinoid Hyperemesis Syndrome," *Federal Practitioner: For the Health Care Professionals of the VA, DoD, and PHS* 34, no. 10 (2017): 33–36, https://www.ncbi.nlm.nih.gov/pmc/articles/PMC6370410/.

30 Sorensen et al., "Cannabinoid Hyperemesis Syndrome."

31 George Sam Wang et al., "Changes in Emergency Department Encounters for Vomiting after Cannabis Legalization in Colorado," *JAMA Network Open* 4, no. 9 (September 2021), https://doi.org/10.1001/jamanetworkopen.2021.25063.

Randy Michael came home for Christmas in 2018. While our visit was pleasant overall, we noticed he was also grappling with inner turmoil, and he grew more agitated and irrational after he had been home for a few days. We didn't know it at the time, but we have learned that marijuana users start to feel heightened effects of withdrawal after about three to five days of not using. Anxiety increases and sleep can become difficult at that time.

On multiple occasions during Randy Michael's visits, I would stumble upon vape pens or lighters, especially on the couch. He told me they were for nicotine. Naively, I believed him, hopping on that river of denial. I wish that I would have recognized that he was using them for high-potency THC cartridges.

You Need to Know

Although proponents of marijuana often claim it is not addictive, more recent research shows that it often is.[32] Much depends on the potency of the product and how often it is being used.[33]

Other studies show that common withdrawal symptoms, which peak around two to six days of not using, include anxiety, irritability, anger, aggression, disturbed sleep/dreaming, depressed mood, and loss of appetite. Less common physical signs are chills, headaches, physical tension, sweating, and stomach pain.[34]

---

[32] Amna Zehra et al., "Cannabis Addiction and the Brain: A Review," *Journal of Neuroimmune Pharmacology* 13 (March 2018): 438–52, https://doi.org/10.1007/s11481-018-9782-9.

[33] National Institute on Drug Abuse, "Is Marijuana Addictive?," April 13, 2021, https://nida.nih.gov/publications/research-reports/marijuana/marijuana-addictive.

[34] Jason P. Connor et al., "Clinical Management of Cannabis Withdrawal," *Addiction* 117, no. 7 (2022): 2075–95, https://doi.org/10.1111/add.15743.

> Although the withdrawal symptoms are not as physically intense as those from opioids or other drugs, they can be emotionally and psychologically overwhelming. Because THC is stored in fat cells, as the body continues to metabolize the fat cells, the withdrawal symptoms can last longer compared to other drugs; some studies suggest up to a month or longer.[35]

Upon returning to Boulder after Christmas, still in his gap year, Randy Michael got a job that started in the spring of 2019 as a leasing agent for a property management company. He loved the new job and was enthusiastic about his work, which not only offered him a better income but also provided a more dynamic and enjoyable atmosphere than his bank job. In June, he moved into a rented home with a couple of University of Colorado–Boulder students, embracing the change and the convenience of living near campus. He seemed content.

In June 2019, he returned home for his father's fiftieth birthday, which we were planning to celebrate with a big party in the backyard. When we asked Randy Michael to assist with some light outdoor chores, he sat down on a bench in our back entry, started crying inconsolably, and carried on. We could not understand what was going on or why he was so upset and agitated.

"I am going to leave and go stay in a hotel," he abruptly declared before heading off on his bike, carrying only a small drawstring backpack. When he returned a few hours later, he was content and calm—a totally different person.

Looking back, I am confident Randy Michael pedaled off to obtain some marijuana, although I didn't consider that possibility

---

[35] Udo Bonnet and Ulrich W. Preuss, "The Cannabis Withdrawal Syndrome: Current Insights," *Substance Abuse and Rehabilitation* 8 (April 2017): 9–37, https://doi.org/10.2147/SAR.S109576.

at the time. (As a good friend often says, "The river of 'De—nial' is long.") Today, we think Randy Michael likely traveled home without drugs, believing he could manage without them, but after a few days he would grow so distressed and irrational that he would have to seek out his next fix.

Outward Signs of Progress

In August 2019, Randy and I visited Randy Michael in Boulder for about three days. It turned out to be a wonderful and uneventful trip. We were delighted to accompany our son as he graciously guided us to his cherished spots in and around Boulder, took us to dinner with one of his friends, treated us to his favorite cookie place, played UNO by the pool at our hotel, and even gave us a tour of his workplace.

Randy Michael appeared to be doing well, and we felt immensely proud of him. Although he openly acknowledged his marijuana use and partying, it seemed he had found a way to manage his life, so we respected his independence and did not battle over behavior we disagreed with. He was entirely self-reliant—apart from our paying for his phone service—a rare accomplishment for any nineteen-year-old in today's world.

He returned home later that month, and the three of us visited the Minnesota State Fair. He embraced our time there with childlike joy, playing arcade games, and convincing me to join him on a roller coaster. I reluctantly accepted his invitation, and now cherish what was our last amusement park ride together. He also excelled at a pull-up challenge, showcasing his dedication to working out. I treasure a photo we made at dusk that day where Randy Michael appears to be holding the giant neon Ferris wheel.

That fall, Randy Michael became a Colorado resident, enabling him to benefit from in-state tuition. He completed the necessary paperwork to enroll at Longmont Community College, including the financial aid applications. Although he was independent of us, he was still under twenty-four, so we were required to disclose our family's financial information so he could access financial aid or grants.

When he saw that information, Randy Michael became agitated and demanded that we fund his college education entirely. We told him we would not financially support his education if he chose to use marijuana, and he declared we were not allowing him to lead a "normal" life involving marijuana use. We stuck to our boundaries, which frustrated him greatly.

Inner Signs of Trouble

He called home one morning that fall to tell us he had been laid off from his leasing job, citing a slowdown in business and a reduced need for apartment clean-outs because it was the beginning of the academic year. We believed his explanation—with students arriving and settling in for the new school year ahead. We worried about his lack of income, but he quickly secured a new leasing agent position with a different property management company in the Boulder area.

However, after Randy Michael's death, we discovered from his journal entries that he had been fired—not laid off—and that he most likely lost his job because of what we now believe was his first psychotic episode.

You Need to Know

People in psychosis experience delusions and false beliefs. They may believe people are sending them special messages or can read their minds, or think other people are trying to hurt them. Some people with psychosis also experience hallucinations—seeing visions or hearing sounds or voices. Sometimes they exhibit inappropriate behavior or speak incoherently.

Although we would not know it until later, Randy Michael began journaling on his computer in the fall of 2019. When we read the entries after his death, we discovered we had not been seeing a full picture of our son or what he was experiencing. I include some of those journal entries in the coming pages because they show in his own words his inner turmoil and his emotional and mental deterioration.

October 2019

I honestly really miss working for "Five Constellations." I thought for some dumb fucking reason that they were part of the mob. I miss working for them, and honestly, showings are really the only thing outside of the free time that I have right now that I enjoy about my current job. I thought they were part of the mob because I was so fucked up this summer. I am doubtful they will consider me, but I am so interested in the position. I guess we will see. . . .

When we visited Randy Michael in August 2019, we were pleasantly surprised by his apparent well-being. It's unsettling now to realize how much he might have been struggling during our visit. Perhaps the onset of his psychosis occurred after our departure? His journals suggest his psychosis emerged in the fall of 2019, and he also documented thoughts of suicide shortly thereafter, although he had appeared content and happy during our visit.

It baffles me how well he managed to mask his internal turmoil with his charm and big smile. Sadly, we have learned that he was a very good actor because we never saw the turmoil that his journal entries from that period revealed, and we learned that psychosis can be subtle. Forty to sixty percent of the time a person suffering might appear to hold it all together, but inside they are falling apart.

October 12, 2019

I used to know what I wanted, a pretty girl, a good-paying job, and friends.

Now I am lost. I don't know what I want and if I even want to be here. Yeah, life could be worse, but it also could be better.

I wish that I could have certain things I'll never have, and honestly, a lot of days, I wish I had a gun I could just put to my head. Everyone around me seems smarter or like they are in some loop that I'm not, and I would say it's beginning to get on my nerves, but it has been like this for a while. Last night I went to smoke, and luckily the bowl was ashed. I literally got nothing, no high. None. But I think those watching me thought I did because one friend with them ignored me and another got too high, ironically. I just am sort of sick of this. I hate my past, and if I had some of the knowledge I do now, I would probably be with 1 of the two girls I have fallen for in my life. I would say I don't care about that anymore, but it really bothers me because that's not me anymore, and who knows if they know about all of this Illuminati shit happening. I've felt mentally unhappy for a long time since I was like 15. But at least before, I was able to use drugs to mask that. Now, I'm back to the same old me. I don't think I'll ever find a woman that I'd wanna spend the rest of my life with because even if someone was very compatible, I don't know if I would be able to trust they are who they say they are. At the end of the day, all I wanted was a family, more importantly, the opportunity to raise children. What am I doing. 90% of my friends I think are fake. Everyone besides "Mike," "Joe," and "Patrick." I wish "Trey" was actually my friend, but like "James," I think that he was a friend out of force or pity, which sucks because I really like him and appreciate his efforts to help normalize me. I just wanna be the best, and I don't know if there is enough time in the day for that. I wish I didn't have to work so much so that I could pursue new ideas and knowledge and really do what I want. I also wish I was still working with "Five Constellations" because I am 85% sure they are involved in the drug trade. I just get so sick and tired of doing this. I wish I had love, something to really be proud of and prove others wrong, or something to be respected for. I lack all of these things. I think my mom loves me, but she doesn't even know the real me, and I think my dad loves me out of guilt or something. My sisters would be sad if I died, as would many people. But when it comes to the reality, they really don't love me. The only love I've felt has either been one-sided or from a substance these last few years. Sometimes, actually, a lot. I wish that branch would have held tight to that belt around my neck or that life would give me a reason to not feel that way. Idk I hope things get better one day. I hope to find better things.

October 15, 2019

I still feel pretty lost. I tried smoking weed last night and when I was at "Five Constellations," these two people came and asked me a million questions and corrected me on what I was doing wrong. Maybe they only talk to me when I'm high. I don't know if I wanna keep taking classes or just start working and taking real estate classes. I'm at a crossroads once again. Idk if I'll even be able to get into Leeds. I keep going back and forward in my head about "Lisa," and even tho I haven't seen her in a year, I have realized I am in no way over her. I just want to find a girl to hang out and fuck with to get my mind away from Lisa. It's kind of killing me. I think "Andy" is pretty fake. It's hard to tell. He agrees with everything I say and says me too to all of it, and I'm just super confused. I thought I was doing right by not smoking but I want to see if it's allowed here and there. I know ur not supposed to get that high because of how celebrities smoke. They just puff out huge clouds and smoke at first. I kind of wanted to try that tn with that cute girl, but it seemed like she and that guy had to go. I'm still lost with everything people were doing to me this summer. Idk. I find it hard to stay soberly motivated and feel like I'm always overthinking. I just feel like my self-worth is less and less every month. I feel like a freak like I can't relate, I want to pursue girls more, but I am so worried they are just testing me. I wish I wouldn't have been so stressed at the gas station the other day when I helped those girls pay for their food—both of them were gorgeous. Idk. All of this is making me feel like a wreck.

If anyone is still reading what I'm saying. Please help me. I'm not well.

Gonna not smoke tomorrow. Enjoy a book for the evening. I like the (almost) final project for "Thor."

These journal entries show Randy Michael could have been dealing with schizophrenia, a disorder that affects a person's ability to perceive, think, feel, and behave clearly.[36] His writing shows that he perceived other people as being inauthentic and that he was experiencing depersonalization and dealing with suicidal thoughts. It's also likely that the two people who "came and asked me a million questions" were hallucinations. All these symptoms could be signs of cannabis-induced psychosis.[37] The

---

36 Shweta Patel et al., "The Association Between Cannabis Use and Schizophrenia: Causative or Curative? A Systematic Review," *Cureus* 12, no. 7 (July 21, 2020), https://doi.org/10.7759/cureus.9309.

37 M. Arendt et al., "Cannabis-Induced Psychosis and Subsequent Schizophrenia Spectrum Disorders: Follow-Up Study of 535 Incident Cases," *British Journal of Psychiatry* 187 (2005): 510–15, https://doi.org/10.1192/bjp.187.6.510.

link between cannabis use and the onset of schizophrenia has been published in several studies.[38]

> ### *You Need to Know*
>
> Almost 50 percent of individuals who experience an initial episode of cannabis-induced psychosis are diagnosed with schizophrenia two to four years after their first psychosis experience.[39] The onset of schizophrenia is approximately ten years earlier for those who are regular cannabis users versus those who are not.[40]

---

38 M. Di Forti et al., "The Contribution of Cannabis Uses to Variation in the Incidence of Psychotic Disorders across Europe (EU-GEI): A Multicentre Case-Control Study," *Lancet* 6, no. 5 (2019):427–36, https://doi.org/10.1016/S2215-0366(19)30048-3.

39 M. Starzer, M. Nordentoft, and C. Hjorthoj, "Rates and Predictors of Conversion to Schizophrenia or Bipolar Disorder following Substance-Induced Psychosis," *American Journal of Psychiatry,* 175, no. 4 (2018): 343–50, https://doi.org/10.1176/appi.ajp.2017.17020223.

40 Arendt et al., "Cannabis-Induced Psychosis."

CHAPTER 7

HOPEFUL LOVE

Signs of Progress—And a Pandemic

In November 2019, we took all four kids on a family vacation during the Thanksgiving holiday. We spent a few days in Boulder and then headed to Steamboat Springs. I let Randy Michael know when we arrived in Boulder, but he said he was spending the day with friends. We had not seen him since September, so I was sad and disappointed that he chose to stay with his friends over getting together with us once we arrived.

Randy Michael had to work the next day, but we had dinner together and accompanied him to collect the new ski boots that we had bought him for his twentieth birthday. Our early Thanksgiving morning drive to Steamboat Springs was serene. We purchased Starbucks on the road, and the kids were laughing and chatting, happily anticipating a couple of fun days together.

The next few days were filled with walks, movies, card games, relaxing dinners, and exploring the area near our condo. Although snowfall in the area was modest, Randy Michael relished a day of skiing, and he exhibited absolutely no signs of suicidal or psychotic behavior for the whole trip. It truly was a most cherished Thanksgiving holiday for all of us.

Because Randy Michael had to work on Sunday afternoon, he caught an early shuttle back to Boulder while the rest of us drove back separately. Before departing for the airport, we stopped by his office to bid farewell, leaving him with our surplus food and water. Relishing our amazing vacation, we eagerly anticipated reuniting at Christmas.

(Mostly) Joyful Christmas

Randy Michael came home for Christmas a few weeks later, and as usual, I hosted the day for my side of our family. I was oddly emotional that day, somehow sensing it might be our final family gathering with everyone together. At the time, I was mostly concerned about my aging parents. I did not suspect it would be the last time we would celebrate Christmas with our young son.

Overall, this holiday visit went well, although Randy Michael became very argumentative a few times. One eruption came on Christmas Day.

Because we were uncertain about Randy Michael's substance use, we did not allow him to use our cars when he was home. On Christmas Day, he came into the kitchen and asked, "Hey, can I go to the casino with 'Joe'?"

Reluctant to spark a confrontation, we tried to avoid answering. He continued to press until we said no. Then he attempted to persuade Sabrina to drive him to St. Paul to grab his friend and then to drive to the casino in a distant suburb, roughly forty minutes away. We decided that we were not going to allow this outing on Christmas Day, even if Sabrina agreed to drive him.

Randy Michael kept pressing the issue as his frustration and anger escalated until he was yelling, "Fuck you! You are so controlling. . . . You just don't want me to have any fun. . . . You never let me do anything. . . . Go fuck yourself, Sabrina!"

His disrespectful outburst in front of our extended family members and younger cousins left me shaky, shocked, and embarrassed. I apologized to our wide-eyed family, confused by why Randy Michael would have such an urgent need to be at the casino on Christmas Day. Today, I can see that his irrational behavior most likely stemmed from the effects of cannabis withdrawal[41] and his addiction.

A few days after Christmas, Randy Michael and I sat together on the couch and dove into another heartfelt conversation about marijuana. He felt we had derailed his life by restricting his marijuana use and limiting our financial support for him because of his use. I told him that one of our goals as parents was to impart our values to our children, but as adults we also know that he is free to choose his own values. I shared that we don't value marijuana use because of its potential for addiction and its negative impact on his life. Therefore, we don't have to support him, because in essence, we would then also be supporting his habit.

Randy Michael again emphasized that he believed marijuana was safe and beneficial, and we both agreed that our values simply did not align. I tried to let him know he had autonomy as an independent individual and asserted that he was free to make his own choices—even when those choices did not align with the values of his parents—and gently suggested that he should explore alternative ways to address his depression and anxiety rather than resorting to marijuana.

No matter how I explained our decisions, Randy Michael was hurt because we would not affirm his marijuana use. He fre-

---

[41] Bonnet and Preuss, "Cannabis Withdrawal Syndrome."

quently described his experiences at wilderness camp and boarding school as damaging and made it clear that he still resented our decisions to send him there. I tried to explain that our decisions had been made with the best intentions in mind and with professional guidance.

It was challenging for Randy Michael to accept perspectives beyond his own convictions, which I believe were rooted in his cannabis use disorder. Because he did not want to quit using marijuana, he relentlessly insisted that it was good for him. It was the lie that his addicted brain convincingly told him and that his addicted brain was happy to believe, as can be seen in a journal entry from about that time.

December 2019

This is my first time being home sober in a long time, and it's starting to make sense. I almost grabbed my weed vape but decided not to last second. I never really put two and two together. I was really struggling for a while. Today we watched family videos for the first time, and I realized that I sort of forced out the majority of childhood memories that I had. My childhood was pretty normal until my freshman and sophomore years. I think I was different from most kids at school, and I just wanted to be liked. I was going about it in the wrong way. Then sophomore year came, and most friends, besides Aaron, sort of shut me out of their friend groups. I felt depressed as I really liked being social at the time. I started smoking pot a little bit because it felt good, and it was what some of my good older friends were doing, but they had all gone to college, and I was alone with few friends. I had gotten caught freshman year summer, and my parents disowned me for a month, and that was the end of that summer. I came into my sophomore year having not hung out with anyone for such a long time. I was alone for most of my 1st semester. I really liked getting high because it took away my social angst and made me feel comfortable all of the time. I started smoking again because I had ordered a vaporizer right before I got caught that summer because I hated regular smoking (coughing part) at the time. I realized that I liked being high all of the time over Christmas break once I picked up weed again. Then the 1st day back to school, I got high and felt good; combined with my ADHD medicine, it made the time go by fast and class (which I usually hated) more enjoyable. I also started to fit in with the cool kids as I was much more chill, and girls started taking notice of me more, too (as I was very popular as a class clown in middle school). It felt good to be like this again. I was getting back into art more and had more friends. Then in about April, Aaron killed himself, I partially blamed myself for this, and I couldn't fully forgive myself for being high when he called to talk to me. I told him we should talk when we game later that night as we did most nights. The following day I woke up to find out he was dead. My best friend at the time took his life, and I smoked the pain away, but not for good. I then had a very socially active summer.

This journal entry sheds so much light on how and why Randy Michael began using marijuana. He turned to marijuana seeking social acceptance and a sense of comfort, as he was grappling with guilt over the loss of his friend, among numerous other challenges. It is evident from this writing that he used weed consistently from the age of sixteen, vaping high-potency products, and was easily hooked.

> ### You Need to Know
>
> As marijuana is legalized in more and more states, more and more young people believe it is safe.[42] They often begin to use marijuana because someone near and dear to them suggests that they try it, and they typically get the product from someone close to them.[43] Vaping provides a way to use highly potent THC products, while its odorless output helps to avoid detection. The range in potency can range from 30 percent to 99 percent THC. The higher the potency, the more detrimental to the developing brain.[44]

Love First

We had another intense argument with Randy Michael before heading to Mass on the Feast of the Holy Family the weekend after Christmas. Once again, he was adamant that we owed him, and he deserved to have his college paid for. Interestingly, our priest's sermon centered on family dynamics, and he emphasized the importance of choosing to prioritize family relationships despite disagreements. Choosing the person over the situation demonstrates unconditional love, he said.

Following Mass and that homily, both Randy Michael and I seemed to settle down. Over a nice dinner, we delved into the

---

42 L. D. Johnston et al., *Monitoring the Future National Survey Results on Drug Use 1975–2016: Overview, Key Findings on Adolescent Drug Use* (Ann Arbor: Institute for Social Research, The University of Michigan, 2017), https://monitoringthefuture.org/wp-content/uploads/2022/08/mtf-overview2016.pdf.

43 Scott T. Leatherdale et al., "Youth Perception of Difficulty Accessing Cannabis following Cannabis Legalization and during the Early and Ongoing Stages of the COVID-19 Pandemic: Repeat Cross-Sectional and Longitudinal Data from the COMPASS Study," *Archives of Public Health* 81 (December 15, 2023), https://doi.org/10.1186/s13690-023-01224-x.

44 D. E. Mandelbaum and S. M. de la Monte, "Adverse Structural and Functional Effects of Marijuana on the Brain: Evidence Reviewed," *Pediatric Neurology* 66 (January 2017): 12–20, https://doi.org/10.1016/j.pediatrneurol.2016.09.004.

underlying issues that troubled him, sharing our perspectives openly. It was a cathartic moment, and he seemed to depart with a better understanding that our love and support for him remained unwavering despite our differing values and beliefs.

It felt like a divine intervention—the Holy Spirit working through the priest's message—to bring serenity, harmony, and understanding to both of us and to ease our emotions at that last dinner before he headed back to Colorado.

Although we witnessed some angry eruptions from Randy Michael during his visit home, we heard no talk of suicide and witnessed no signs of psychosis. Instead, we ended that holiday visit reassured by moments of connection and understanding despite the complexities of our differences.

New Year, Fresh Start

In the first couple of months of 2020, Randy Michael enrolled in community college and committed to a regular workout routine. He was attempting what he later described as a "tolerance break" or "T-break." This is when a regular user seeks to stay sober for just a short period of time looking to lower their tolerance and to be able to have that "high and euphoric feeling" once again.

Randy Michael's decision to take a T-break shows he was aware that his mental state wasn't at its best and that he needed to prioritize his fitness and well-being. To achieve this, he focused on his online studies, work commitments, nutrition, and exercise routine. Studies about T-breaks show they are a reason for concern.[45] People who use cannabis and take T-breaks are at greater risk for problematic cannabis use. The study cited shows that

---

45 E. B. Ansell et al., "Cannabis Use Breaks in Young Adults: The Highs and Lows of Tolerance Breaks," *Drug and Alcohol Dependence* 249 (August 2023), https://doi.org/10.1016/j.drugalcdep.2023.109951.

T-breaks are indicative of a need for intervention and prevention. We didn't know it at the time, but Randy Michael definitely needed intervention.

During those T-breaks, Randy Michael frequently phoned me to talk while he prepared his dinner, which was usually chicken and vegetables with rice. We talked about where he was grocery shopping and what his workout routine was like. He had started practicing yoga and volunteering at the studio, enabling him to get a discount for his classes.

He appeared to be managing his life well while maintaining a full course load at the community college and holding down a full-time job in property management. Feeling proud of his efforts and his accomplishments, we came to a new arrangement concerning his tuition. He would cover his tuition expenses up front, and if he achieved As and Bs by the end of the semester, we would reimburse him. He seemed content with this arrangement, and his journal entries reflect Randy Michael's personal insights during this time.

January 2020

Too paranoid. Done w/ drugs. Meditate before I go out. Fuck it. Done with this. Done with making mistakes.

February 2020

It's not that I can't go out sober; it's just that I Begin to get bored very quickly without a buzz or boost in social productivity, which I would expect you to find as being bad.

The World Shifts

In March 2020, as most of us remember, a novel coronavirus upended the world. COVID-19 and the public health restrictions enacted to battle its spread ushered us all into an unprecedented and unsettling period marked by uncertainty and seclusion. Randy Michael had been living with two roommates, both students at CU-Boulder, but they moved back home, leaving him in total isolation. Although his job required him to be "in office," he worked all alone.

Aiming to provide interaction and support, we frequently checked in via FaceTime and set up virtual events to help support Brooke and Randy Michael, who were both living out of state and in seclusion. We initiated virtual "dress-up" dinners, choosing themes for our menu and wardrobe as we cooked and dined together with friends and family over Zoom. One evening, Randy Michael transformed into Elton John for a music-themed dinner.

Throughout the initial weeks of the pandemic lockdown, Randy Michael appeared in good spirits and insisted he was maintaining a schedule and routine. However, he was unable to access the gym or pursue his yoga practice at the studio. The Boulder weather was not conducive to outdoor exercise and by April, he was getting frustrated and lonesome, contacting me multiple times a day—probably as an attempt to make up for his limited social interactions.

He maintained his workout regimen by investing in an exercise bike and free weights, aiming to get "ripped" for the summer, as revealed in his journal.

April 2020

21-day cut 1800–1900 cal (RAPID FAT LOSS)

Get shredded for summer

Drink a bottle of water

Every morning (50 push-ups)—if shoulders are lacking, like me

30 min light bike ride/walk

10 min of HIT core

Shoulders

Rest (2.5–4.5 mile run)

Biceps + triceps

Rest (2.5–4.5 mile run)

Chest + back

Rest (2.5–4.5 mile run)

Repeat

Intermittent fasting 12 pm–8 pm

Total g of protein 160–200 a day

12–2 pm:

Banana 120 c

whey shake 3 scoops 420 cal

540 cal

Protein (75g)

+3 eggs

(225 cal)

21g protein

2–5 pm:

Protein bar 1x200 cal

20g of protein

6–9 pm:

Dinner meat x veggies (high density long-lasting carbs)

200–300 cal of chicken breast or ground turkey

10–20g of protein

100–200 cal of veggies (mixed veggies, crushed cauliflower, pasta sauce, mixed fried rice-) *NO OIL

—as much salt as you want 😀

Total 300–600 cal

8–10 pm

2–3x scoops of whey protein

420 cal

NO FOOD TILL 12 pm TOMORROW (go into brief ketosis)

ONCE Gyms are open again, add leg day, 300–500 cal to the deficit, and cut out cardio plus push-ups if you want. This will help gain back muscle mass and maintain definition

Tips- DRINK a ton of water

Good luck & F*ck the government for shutting everything down . . .

When I read this, my heart breaks. He was trying so hard!

In late April or early May, Randy Michael told us he was considering buying a motorcycle. I started praying that he would not. He had little to no riding experience and lived in the mountains, which we felt increased a motorcycle's inherent risks. Despite our concerns, we attempted to be supportive when he called to share his excitement about finally acquiring the bike. We knew he was alone in a world turned upside down, and we hoped the motorcycle would bring him some happiness.

With no end in sight to the uncertainty surrounding COVID, Randy and I grew more apprehensive about Randy Michael's situation in Boulder. Brooke had temporarily returned home from Texas; she could work remotely, but Randy Michael didn't have that option and we knew he was lonely.

Randy visited our son over Memorial Day weekend and said Boulder was a ghost town. Everything was deserted or closed to the public. But the visit did give him a chance to teach Randy Michael the basics of safe motorcycle riding in an empty parking lot near the Boulder campus. I was relieved knowing Randy Michael had received a few lessons from his dad and happy when he successfully passed his motorcycle licensing test when the DMV eventually reopened. As a result of Randy's visit, our sweet son sent the following email to his dad.

May 25, 2020

Hey dad,
It was really great having you out here this weekend. With everything going on it has been very lonely, depressing, and difficult. I think you coming out here was what I really needed. I am so grateful that you are my father and cherish all of the times we have had in my heart. From listening to nickleback in the vet to hockey games with you, I have been blessed to have you as a father figure in my life. With all of the uncertainty in the world right now it is nice to know that we still have a meaningful relationship. I wish I would have taken our time together more seriously during the last few difficult years that I caused living with you guys. I was lost and needed to figure out some things on my own. I still kind of am lost and know that I have a lot to figure out. I have faith that things will go the way they are supposed to and wanted you to know that I hope that we can see each other more! You are a great man and it makes me sad to split up again. I hope you fly safe and give mom a

hug for me. I thought about writing you a letter, but digital ink is forever ;) I love you and I hope you know if anything happens to me that I am very grateful for the time that we have gotten to spend together. Kick ass in real estate this upcoming season.

Love, Little Guy!

Randy Michael references not seeing his dad here again, but we attributed it to the uncertainty in the world, not suicidal ideation. So insightful that digital ink is forever, and we will forever treasure emails like this one.

CHAPTER 8

HELPLESS AND HEARTBREAKING LOVE

Slow yet Steady Decline

In June 2020, Randy Michael came home to help celebrate my fiftieth birthday, and it turned out to be one of our most wonderful visits. He appeared serene, content, optimistic, and in good spirits, full of jokes and lighthearted, and he wrote me the sweetest birthday card, which you can see in Figure 8.1.

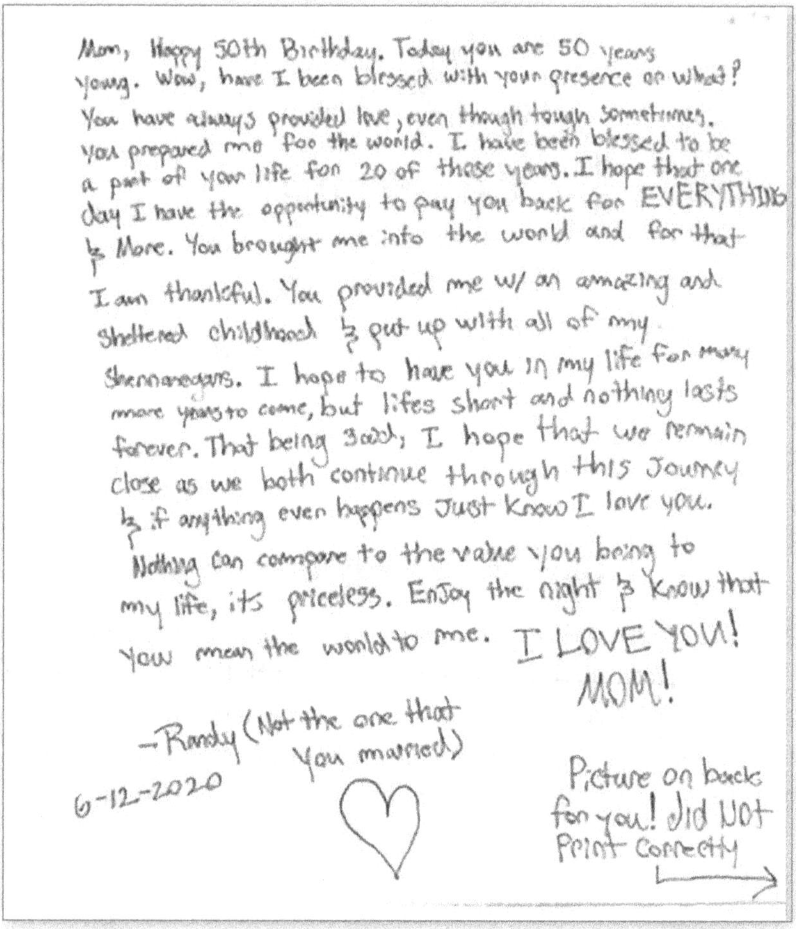

> Mom, Happy 50th Birthday. Today you are 50 years young. Wow, have I been blessed with your presence or what? You have always provided love, even though tough sometimes. You prepared me for the world. I have been blessed to be a part of your life for 20 of these years. I hope that one day I have the opportunity to pay you back for EVERYTHING & More. You brought me into the world and for that I am thankful. You provided me w/ an amazing and sheltered childhood & put up with all of my shenanagans. I hope to have you in my life for many more years to come, but lifes short and nothing lasts forever. That being said, I hope that we remain close as we both continue through this journey & if anything even happens just know I love you. Nothing can compare to the value you being to my life, its priceless. Enjoy the night & know that you mean the world to me. I LOVE YOU! MOM!
>
> —Randy (Not the one that you married)
> 6-12-2020
>
> Picture on back for you! Did NOT print correctly →

Figure 8.1. Randy Michael wrote a sweet—and slightly chilling—note for my birthday.

I treasure this card. It hangs in my office and helps me feel his love every day.

His note warmed my heart, yet his allusion to the brevity of life also unsettled me a bit. However, it did not seem too strange because all our kids are acutely aware that their father lost his whole family when he was seventeen. We opt to say, "I love you," more often than not, aware that life is filled with uncertainties. I chalked up the odd reference to our family history.

Unlike many of Randy Michael's recent visits, this one was uneventful. He mentioned having new roommates in Boulder and said he disliked one named "Tom" because he was "strange." He said Tom watched him and took his things. I assumed it was simply a personality clash. Only later did I realize his complaints about Tom could have been signs of Randy Michael's growing paranoia.

During his stay, I made a point to tell Randy Michael how proud I was that he had managed his life so well the past few months during the isolation and challenges of the COVID pandemic. When he left, the whole family agreed that Randy Michael seemed to be in better shape than he had been in a long time and that it was our best visit ever.

Although COVID canceled our usual late summer trip to the Minnesota State Fair, Randy Michael came home over Labor Day weekend. We had another pleasant visit, and he seemed content, happy, and unusually calm.

Randy Michael loved discussing various topics—health, politics, world events, spirituality, AI, real estate, clothing, investing—you name it. One afternoon during his Labor Day visit, he came up to my office to chat. I can vividly picture him sitting across from me at my desk, his hair styled short on the sides, line cut with a longer top, sporting a handsome smile, wearing the flowered shirt I had bought him earlier in the summer for our family photos. He enthusiastically detailed his new ventures in web design consulting and ideas for his own clothing business although he seemed more contemplative than usual. We explored several facets of our family, his work, and his aspirations during that conversation.

Randy Michael floated the idea of taking time off from school after intense spring and summer semesters juggling full-time work and online classes and creating two businesses—all while in isolation. I encouraged him to continue classes, but he didn't seem inclined to do so. He also hinted at quitting his job as a leasing agent, and I suggested he should find another job first. I again expressed my pride at how well he was handling the trials that characterized life in 2020 and told him I sensed a change in his demeanor, a shift that I had seen since early spring.

> ### *Hindsight*
>
> I credit maternal instinct for detecting a shift in Randy Michael in the fall of 2020. Although my instinct was not entirely off base, it was not finely tuned enough to detect what was really happening to my son. Now I know that early onset and frequent use of high-potency marijuana products was the catalyst that transformed Randy Michael's thinking, perception, personality, and cognitive functions.[46] It structurally reshaped his brain, leading to irrational thinking, depression, anxiety, psychosis, and suicidal thoughts.[47, 48]

In that office conversation, Randy Michael confided in me about a series of distressing thoughts and dreams that had plagued him in the spring, when he said he had been trying to

---

46 Emese Kroon et al., "Heavy Cannabis Use, Dependence and the Brain: A Clinical Perspective," *Addiction* 115, no. 3 (2020): 559–72, https://doi.org/10.1111/add.14776.

47 Lawrence M. Scheier and Kenneth W. Griffin, "Youth Marijuana Use: A Review of Causes and Consequences," *Current Opinion in Psychology* 38 (2021): 11–18, https://doi.org/10.1016/j.copsyc.2020.06.007.

48 K. C. Winters and H. Waldron, "An Examination of the Association between Cannabis and Psychosis," in *Essays on Adolescent Health*, ed. S. Satel and N. Riley (Washington, DC: American Enterprise Institute, forthcoming).

exercise and cut down on marijuana use. But he also mentioned trying psychoactive mushrooms, perhaps to find solace amid the upsetting thoughts and dreams.

"Mom, I have talked with God and the Devil. No one is 100 percent good or 100 percent bad," he said. "Everyone's a blend of both." I listened, as a mother does, surprised by his revelations.

After detailing some of life's uncertainties he said, "I love you, Mom, no matter what happens. Please know that."

I replied, "You are worrying me, Randy. Are you okay?"

He told me he had occasionally stopped using marijuana but confessed, "I thought that I wanted to kill myself when I wasn't using." This experience made him even more sure that marijuana was his savior.

"Randy, there are better medications intended to help with anxiety and depression if that is what you have," I told him. "Please go to a doctor, someone who knows medications and can help you find the one that works best for you."

Randy Michael assured me that marijuana was all he needed and that he would be okay. The conversation about the benefits of marijuana were like so many conversations we had been having for years—circular and juxtaposed. But that day Randy Michael was calm, philosophical, almost indifferent, exhibiting none of the anger or aggression he had displayed so frequently during those previous discussions.

> ### You Need to Know
>
> Marijuana can rearrange the adolescent brain, affect dopamine production and cognition, and spiral users into cycles of depression, anxiety, paranoia, and psychosis.[49, 50] Some studies show that half of people who experience cannabis-induced psychosis will transition to schizophrenia.[51] In fact, a 2023 Denmark study showed that 30 percent of schizophrenia cases in men ages twenty-one to thirty could have been avoided if they had not experienced cannabis use disorder.[52]

During this particular visit home, Randy Michael once again told us how much he disliked his roommate Tom, saying Tom would casually stroll into the kitchen shirtless, intrude into his room, and help himself to his belongings. Randy Michael told us he had set up a camera in his room to catch Tom in the act while he was visiting us in Minnesota. His descriptions seemed off, and I knew Randy Michael could be difficult to live with and thought maybe he and Tom just didn't get along.

In hindsight, I think Randy Michael was having paranoid thoughts about Tom that were triggered by his frequent use of highly potent marijuana.[53]

---

49 Michael A. P. Bloomfield et al., "The Effects of Δ9-Tetrahydrocannabinol on the Dopamine System," *Nature* 539 (2016): 369–77, https://doi.org/10.1038/nature20153.

50 J. Mennis, G. J. Stahler, and M. Mason, "Cannabis Legalization and the Decline of Cannabis Use Disorder (CUD) Treatment Utilization in the US," *Current Addiction Reports* 10, no. 1 (January 2023): 38–51, https://doi.org/10.1007/s40429-022-00461-4.

51 Gniewko Więckiewicz et al., "Intensity of Psychoactive Substance Use Affects the Occurrence of Prodromal Symptoms of Psychosis," *Journal of Clinical Medicine* 13, no. 3 (January 2024): 760, https://doi.org/10.3390/jcm13030760.

52 Carsten Hjorthøj et al., "Association between Cannabis Use Disorder and Schizophrenia Stronger in Young Males Than in Females," *Psychological Medicine* 53, no. 15 (2023): 7322–28, https://doi.org/10.1017/S0033291723000880.

53 Daniel Freeman et al., "How Cannabis Causes Paranoia: Using the Intravenous Administration of Δ9-Tetrahydrocannabinol (THC) to Identify Key Cognitive Mechanisms Leading to Paranoia," *Schizophrenia Bulletin* 41, no. 2 (2015): 391–99, https://doi.org/10.1093/schbul/sbu098.

We bid each other farewell at the airport on September 7, 2020. Although Randy Michael had been tolerating only one-armed, sideways hugs on his recent visits, this time I insisted he face me, and I enveloped him in a big hug with both arms reaching up to his steep shoulders. Standing on the curb of the Hubert Humphrey Terminal in St. Paul, we held the hug longer than usual, and I can still hear him laughing gently in my ear, saying, "Really, Mom . . . how much longer?"

Over the past three years, whenever Randy Michael departed, I would embrace him tightly and silently recite a Hail Mary in my mind. I was constantly worried for his well-being yet knew he had to navigate his path independently. By invoking the protection of the Virgin Mary, I felt a measure of comfort and peace knowing that something greater than I held my son when I couldn't be by his side.

This time, as I hugged Randy Michael close, I whispered the Hail Mary aloud into his ear, ending with, "He is yours now." As I released him, I explained that I entrusted the Virgin Mary to watch over him from that moment forward. He didn't object; instead, he hugged me back and smiled.

It was the last time I would see my son alive.

The Shadow of Regret

How I wish I could go back in time! If I could rewind the clock, I would never drop him off at the airport. Instead of whispering a Hail Mary in his ear, I would have whispered, "Stay with us. Please, let us help you. I know that you're hurting, and your brain is hijacked."

Looking back now, armed with the wisdom hindsight bestows, I wish I had held on tighter, adamant in my resolve not to let him slip away. I could have reassured him and reminded him of our unwavering support. I should have whisked him to a doctor's office, insisting he get the care that he deserved, the care that he needed. If I had known then what I know now, I'm certain we could have gotten him placed in a treatment and recovery center where healing was possible, where the darkness he was experiencing could have been pierced by light and hope.

Yet amid this torment of regret about what I could or should have done, I cannot ignore the truth that Randy Michael was a young man capable of making his own decisions. He possessed free will and an autonomy we had to respect, even though it would break our hearts.

The cruelest irony is that Randy Michael remained oblivious to the truth that his brain was broken, and that marijuana was the culprit harming him. A staunch advocate for marijuana, he fervently believed it was beneficial for him. Unfortunately, too many young people are suffering because they fail to see how marijuana/THC is harmful to them.[54]

While I refuse to dwell in the shadow of regret, I cannot deny its presence nor its weight upon my heart. In the depths of my being, I still yearn for the warmth of our son's embrace, for the melody of his laughter to grace our days once more.

I can only hope that our journey, our anguish, will serve as a beacon for others who are navigating similar storms.

---

54 A. C. Mariani and A. R. Williams, "Perceived Risk of Harm from Monthly Cannabis Use among US Adolescents: National Survey on Drug Use and Health, 2017," *Preventive Medicine Reports* 23 (September 2021), https://doi.org/10.1016/j.pmedr.2021.101436.

Disconnect in Outer, Inner Lives

When he returned to Boulder, Randy Michael immersed himself in developing his clothing line. He enlisted a childhood friend as a model and hired other acquaintances for photo shoots around Boulder, which he compiled into an impressive video. We were so proud of his work and his boundless creativity.

In October 2020, Randy Michael called to say he had quit his job at the leasing office and was now working at a favorite burrito shop. I couldn't imagine how Randy Michael would sustain himself without a stable income, and I worried when his calls became less and less frequent.

But a few weeks later, he phoned to say he had landed a job at a Nissan dealership, specializing in car sales. We believed he would excel in this role, having witnessed his success setting up new credit card accounts when he worked as a cashier at a retail store in high school. We thought Randy Michael's social charm, motivation for money, and fondness for cars would help him thrive in this job and offer him a chance to make a decent income.

Through phone calls, FaceTime, and texts, we perceived that things were looking up for our son. His journal entries from the time tell a different story.

October 2020

> I still feel pretty lost . . . I don't know if I want to keep taking classes or just start working and taking real estate classes. I'm at a crossroads once again. . . . Idk. I find it hard to stay soberly motivated and feel like I'm always overthinking. I just feel like my self-worth is less and less every month. I feel like a freak like I can't relate.
>
> If anyone is still reading what I'm saying. Please help me. I'm not well.

Randy Michael's journal entries reflect his inner turmoil, detailing suicidal thoughts, depersonalization, disassociation, depression, anxiety, and the grip of addiction. Compounding his distress, he harbored a paranoid belief that someone was reading these deeply personal entries although they were securely stored on his computer.

It is not uncommon for people in cannabis-induced psychosis to think their phones and computers have been hacked and that the whole world might know who they are and what they are doing. In his last months, Randy Michael was certain that people were able to access his computer and his personal information on his phone.

New Job, Old Impulsivity

Transitioning into car sales, Randy Michael became an eager buyer himself as he came across many so-called deals. In October, he purchased a 2005 Mercedes Benz C-Class sedan and then decided to also lease a Nissan Leaf—a much more practical choice with a modest monthly payment.

Shortly after his purchase, issues emerged with the Mercedes, necessitating extensive repairs. Randy Michael swiftly traded it in for a 2004 Corvette with a T-top. He proudly shared details of his purchase with us, but we were worried he would not be able to cover his rent, food, and insurance. We tried to offer guidance from afar, but his drug-influenced decision-making and impaired prefrontal cortex (often referred to as the "seat of second thought") made it hard for him to listen to advice.[55, 56]

---

55 Francesca M. Filbey et al., "Preliminary Findings Demonstrating Latent Effects of Early Adolescent Marijuana Use Onset on Cortical Architecture," *Developmental Cognitive Neuroscience* 16 (2015): 16–22, https://doi.org/10.1016/j.dcn.2015.10.001.

56 Skyler Shollenbarger et al., "Impact of Cannabis Use on Prefrontal and Parietal Cortex Gyrification and Surface Area in Adolescents and Emerging Adults," *Developmental Cognitive Neuroscience* 16 (2015): 46–53, https://doi.org/10.1016/j.dcn.2015.07.004.

HELPLESS AND HEARTBREAKING LOVE

On November 9, 2020, Randy Michael celebrated his twenty-first birthday. There's often parental concern surrounding such milestones. When I talked with him, I asked, "How are you going to celebrate your birthday this evening?"

"I am going out with friends for a few drinks," he told me.

That seemed reasonable to me, given all we had been through with him, so I reminded him of the advice from my favorite workout instructor: "If you can't be good, be careful."

He laughed and assured me he would be good and then asked for a ski pass for his birthday. We happily purchased it for him, anticipating our son enjoying an exciting ski season.

Randy Michael enjoyed selling cars and was upbeat and positive about meeting his sales goals. He shared a video he created for a contest to promote the Nissan Rogue, and he never missed an opportunity to pitch a Nissan Rogue to us! In the video he was articulate, descriptive, dressed in professional attire, and appeared to be doing so well! Although we were proud of his success, we were very disappointed when we discovered that he would not be able to take time from work and visit during Thanksgiving as he was the newest sales team member.

As November faded into December, Randy Michael's calls home became further and further apart. Although we offered to fly him home for Christmas, he said the holidays were hectic, and he would not be able to take time off. Wanting to ensure he felt loved and missed, I sent him a present and home-baked goods each week throughout the month. Randy Michael appreciated each gesture, eagerly anticipating the boxes of goodies and gifts.

On Christmas morning, we connected with Randy Michael via FaceTime. He was skiing solo but mentioned picking up some malt beer for the day. Worried about him drinking and being alone on the mountain, I asked if we could install a location-sharing app on his phone. Surprisingly, he agreed.

CHAPTER 9

UNCONDITIONAL LOVE

Paranoia and Chaos in Denver

In January 2020, no one expected that the whole world would soon be swept up into chaos by a pandemic. Just a year later, our family was engulfed in its own turmoil upending our lives as profoundly as COVID-19 had disrupted the world.

As 2021 began, Randy Michael's calls and texts became increasingly sporadic. We offered to visit him in January, but he said he was going skiing with friends on our proposed dates. Next, we invited him to join us on a trip to Florida in February; he seemed interested but did not commit.

I checked in on him using Life 360, a location-sharing app, and noticed erratic patterns. He would charge his car at the dealership where he worked, but rather than during the day or normal business hours, he'd do it late at night. He was making frequent commutes between Boulder where he was currently living and various locations surrounding Denver. His whereabouts seemed scattered. Occasionally, he would call me late in the evening from a car-charging station. Although our conversations seemed normal, I was concerned about his haphazard schedule.

In mid-January, he called to tell me he had abruptly quit his job at the car dealership, saying the final straw came when a coworker placed a sheet of paper containing strange messages on his desk. Earlier that month, Randy Michael had said this same coworker was giving him dirty looks.

"Mom, this guy looks at me funny every time I use the restroom, or he comes out of the restroom."

I asked Randy Michael to send me a photo of the paper with the "strange messages" and discovered it was merely a flier for someone involved in website development. I told him I thought the coworker was likely trying to be supportive of Randy Michael's side job in the same field. However, Randy Michael's paranoia was escalating, causing him to interpret kind gestures as sinister or antagonistic, and leaving him increasingly distressed, as evidenced by journal entries like this one.

January 2021

Look, God. I am so sorry for real. Like, I feel so shitty inside that I messed up last night. Tbh, I knew I could have been pushing boundaries and taking a risk. . . . Can you please forgive me? Please. I just honestly was dumb for having more than one beer and a Zyn. I honestly feel really bad. But, like am really sorry. I'm not gonna drink anything tn and am going to try and remain completely dry. No nicotine and no alcohol going forward. Please give me this chance. I'm so sick of being alone and just tired of doing this. . . . Please forgive me. Please. I really feel shitty. I'm gonna get rid of my wine and what not too. Idk if you're making fun of me with those people outside, but I'm so sorry. I know I have said it before, but I just wanna start doing the right thing, and it was dumb to even tempt myself. I'm really done this time.

As can be seen in this journal entry, Randy Michael was drinking and using Zyns (a nicotine pouch) at this point in his life, in addition to marijuana. Broader substance abuse is common among many marijuana users, especially those who start using marijuana at a young age. Individuals who experience cannabis-induced psychosis often turn to other substances to quiet their minds, seeking relief that marijuana no longer provides.

> ### *You Need to Know*
> Marijuana has been called a gateway drug, but it might be more accurate to call it a "foundation" or "promoter" drug. Per the National Institute on Drug Abuse (NIDA) 2021 report, marijuana use can serve as a stepping stone to other substance use.[57] According to a study published in 2023, youth marijuana users were 5.6 times more likely to use alcohol, 7.9 times more likely to binge drink, 15.8 times more likely to drink heavily, 8.9 times more likely to use cigarettes, and 9.9 times more likely to use illicit drugs.[58]

For the Love of Rap

After Randy Michael quit his dealership job, he announced that he intended to become a "pot-smoking" rap artist. We were dumbfounded; although Randy Michael had always appreciated music, he had never demonstrated any musical talent. We tried to be

---

57 National Institute on Drug Abuse, "Cannabis (Marijuana) Drug Facts," December 24, 2019, https://nida.nih.gov/publications/drugfacts/cannabis-marijuana.

58 Robert L. DuPont, Beth Han, Corinne L. Shea, and Bertha K. Madras, "Drug Use among Youth: National Survey Data Support a Common Liability of All Drug Use," Institute for Behavior and Health (Rockville, MD), McLean Hospital (Belmont, MA), and Harvard Medical School (Boston, MA).

patient and supportive, but we were deeply worried and puzzled by this new development and were hoping it would pass.

Our son had left a job he seemed to love and was clearly suited for because he was convinced that he was destined to be the next Mac Miller. I didn't even know who Mac Miller was, and I regret not doing more research at the time into the performer my son was openly emulating. I am sure my reactions to Randy Michael's newfound career aspirations would have been different if I had realized Mac Miller had died of a drug overdose in 2018 at age twenty-six.

Toward the end of January, we began to realize that Randy Michael wasn't functioning well. He seemed distant and not eager to communicate, but he told us a ski fall that had left him bruised and unable to work out was affecting his demeanor. By the end of the month, we were communicating only sporadically by text.

In one text, he mentioned being involved in an accident in his Nissan Leaf that caused around twelve hundred dollars worth of damage to the front fender. He didn't hit anyone; he just ran into a sign, he said. We knew that he had also crashed his motorcycle earlier in the fall and this time suspected he was driving under the influence. Our suspicion was confirmed after his death when we found video footage of Randy Michael smoking marijuana while behind the wheel of his Corvette. Thank God his vehicle accidents didn't involve anyone else.

You Need to Know

Most experts believe marijuana impairs driving ability, and many have blamed it for an increase in fatal accidents in Washington and Colorado after the states legalized its use. At a minimum, the correlation between increased marijuana use and fatal traffic accidents is concerning.[59, 60]

Hindsight

In some states, like Minnesota, it is possible to look up your loved one's court records. By visiting the Minnesota Court Records Online (MCRO) website, you can search for a name. Almost three years after Randy Michael passed, we discovered that he had been charged with criminal possession of a small amount of marijuana (1.4 grams or more) in his motor vehicle and a moving violation for failure to drive with due care in the neighboring town of Oakdale, Minnesota. These violations occurred about one month before he was to leave for Colorado in July 2018.

Unbeknownst to us, our next-door neighbors, who are attorneys, represented Randy Michael. They were able to plea bargain his charges down to a petty misdemeanor, resulting in a two-hundred-dollar fine and the dismissal of the possession charge on August 10, 2018. He left for Colorado on August 12.

---

59 Brian C. Tefft, Lindsay S. Arnold, and Jurek George Grabowski, *Prevalence of Marijuana Involvement in Fatal Crashes: Washington, 2010–2014* (Washington, DC: AAA Foundation for Traffic Safety, 2016), https://aaafoundation.org/prevalence-marijuana-use-among-drivers-fatal-crashes-washington-2010-2014/.

60 D. T. Myran, A. Gaudreault, M. Pugliese, D. G. Manuel, and P. Tanuseputro, "Cannabis-Involved Traffic Injury Emergency Department Visits after Cannabis Legalization and Commercialization," *JAMA Network Open*, September 6, 2023, https://jamanetwork.com/journals/jamanetworkopen/fullarticle/2808961.

> ### *Hindsight continued:*
> If you're worried about a loved one's potential drug use, checking the court's website might provide information that could confirm your concerns. I wish our neighbors had informed us when Randy Michael got into trouble with the law and displayed risky behavior. While I respect the importance of client confidentiality, I also know these neighbors were well aware of our struggles. This information could have been another sign for us that Randy Michael was on a dangerous path. Unfortunately, for public safety, there is currently no established legal limit for THC use, as there is for alcohol.

One night in late January 2021 Randy Michael called us in distress, sobbing and choking. Eventually he admitted to saying hurtful and horrible things to a childhood friend and he deeply regretted his actions. He also revealed that he had been heavily using marijuana and "micro dosing" magic mushrooms. Randy Michael believed that by taking small amounts of psilocybin (psychedelic mushrooms) and smoking marijuana, he was self-medicating his anxiety and depression by manipulating his serotonin and dopamine levels.

I encouraged Randy Michael to apologize to his friend and find a way to move forward. I also told him we were concerned about his drug use, and he immediately switched from vulnerable and regretful to defensive and irrational. He said he couldn't be honest with me if I kept suggesting that he needed help. Once again, he was unable to regulate or control himself. The human brain is incredibly intricate and altering neurotransmitter levels without professional knowledge—as Randy Michael was doing with his marijuana use and micro dosing—is risky, to say the least. But trying to get someone with a broken, addicted brain to understand that danger is next to impossible.

> ### *You Need to Know*
>
> What is micro dosing? Micro dosing is a way to consume small doses of psychedelics, such as psilocybin ("magic mushrooms") or LSD. Generally, a micro dose is around one-tenth of a recreational dose. Proponents believe that micro dosing may improve mood and focus, increase creativity, and improve overall mental health, but there are not enough studies to back up anecdotal reports. Our youth, however, have ample sources online that make claims on YouTube or other social media platforms touting the "benefits" with no proven scientific evidence.

Headed for Denver

Although Randy Michael was pursuing a "career in rap," he was unemployed, and we did not know how he was going to afford to live. We began regularly tracking his movements on Life 360, and night after night, we could tell that he was cruising around the Denver/Boulder area, visiting various locations at odd hours.

Randy Michael was very resourceful. He moved to Colorado when he was eighteen. The legal age to purchase recreational marijuana in Colorado is twenty-one, but young Randy Michael knew that with a medical marijuana card, he'd legally be able to purchase marijuana sooner. By the time he was nineteen, he had applied for and was granted a medical marijuana card. So, Randy Michael had figured out a way to purchase copious amounts of legal medical marijuana, a product he considered "safe"; how to pay less in taxes; and also sell it locally or ship it to customers/friends outside Colorado, hence supplementing his lifestyle. We speculated he was selling marijuana, but after he passed, we found a screenshot of a Reddit source on his phone that discussed the safest way to ship drugs. Our suspicions were confirmed.

Although we were concerned about his finances and how he was funding his lifestyle, our foremost concern shifted in the next few months to his overall well-being. It was clear that Randy Michael was increasingly dealing with delusions, anger, aggressiveness, and self-destructive behaviors.

Out of touch with reality and certain that he would soon achieve great wealth, our son promised to purchase us a Corvette and a retirement home. I told him what I really wanted was his sobriety. Despite our sincere pleas for his health and wellness, he assured us that he would attain riches and fame. "I will die by trying," he insisted. That statement frightened me even more, but reasoning with him was impossible.

At the end of January, we discovered Randy Michael was moving from Boulder to Denver. He said it was because of ongoing conflicts with his roommate. Unemployed, we had no idea how he could manage such a move, but our ever-resourceful Randy Michael somehow managed to secure a studio apartment in Denver without a job.

He called to tell us about it, excited that he had negotiated a month's rent at no cost. Although he would not tell me the apartment's exact location, he said it was brand-new, boasted a sliding glass door leading out to a charming patio, offered scenic views of the mountains, and was situated near the light rail system in an area undergoing revitalization. In naivety and denial, we were thankful he had a roof over his head and hopeful he would soon be employed.

> ### *Hindsight*
>
> Randy Michael led us to believe that he was choosing to move to Denver, but we later learned that he had been evicted. After his death, I called his Boulder landlord, as I tried to glean any information about our son that I possibly could. Although we had suspected—correctly—that Randy Michael had been evicted, we had no idea why.
>
> The landlord told us he had taken photos of bullets and threatened to use them against his roommates. The behavior was frightening enough to get Randy Michael evicted.
>
> Studies show frequent users of marijuana exhibit violent behavior.[61] If we had known the real reason for Randy Michael's move in 2021, we would have recognized it as another major warning sign that things were amiss, and he wasn't in his right mind.

As we moved through February, Randy Michael flipped from sending occasional messages to bombarding us with text messages, many of them exhibiting extreme paranoia. No matter how carefully I tried to word my responses, he would scrutinize every word, searching for even the slightest hint of criticism. He would then accuse us of lacking support, label us as "fake," and threaten to stop talking with us. It seems his addicted brain was searching for ways to be the victim, to justify his continued and increased marijuana use, and we were the easiest target to continue that vicious cycle.

Randy Michael refused to give me his new address and disabled his location-tracking app, so we had no idea where his new

---

61 Norman S. Miller, Redon Ipeku, and Thersilla Oberbarnscheidt, "A Review of Cases of Marijuana and Violence," *International Journal of Environmental Research and Public Health* 17, no. 5 (February 2020): 1578, https://doi.org/10.3390/ijerph17051578.

apartment was or where he was spending his time. He finally sent me his address when I offered to send him some new pants and a shirt from Lululemon. Knowing where he was living brought a slight sense of relief.

Because of his unpredictable behavior, we decided he should not join us in Florida that year. Randy Michael reached out a few times during our trip and sounded weak and awful on one call. He said he had fallen ill with a stomach bug and asked for advice on how to clean up vomit. He shared that he had thrown up all over his apartment. I suspected his illness was drug-related, but at the time I was not familiar with cannabis hyperemesis syndrome, which we explored in previous chapters.

Our worry for Randy Michael continued to deepen over the next few weeks. In our conversations, he told us he had connected with an audio engineer to fine-tune his music. Knowing he didn't have much musical ability, I worried about people taking advantage of him. When I'd bring it up, he often became agitated and vaguely referenced past traumas, yet refused to discuss specifics. We had no idea what he was recalling. We learned later that this was part of his delusion. He was unable to decipher what was real versus what was not.

He urged us not to disclose his new address to anyone and sometimes talked about severing ties with us so he could focus solely on pursuing his music career. His behavior was so uncharacteristic of who he used to be that I subconsciously began to mourn the loss of our son.

I read his messages again and again and began to speculate whether the trauma he described might have originated from bullying he endured in high school. Perhaps one of the worst occurrences was junior year when he moved out of our home.

Shortly after, some of his "friends" picked him up and drove him to a homeless shelter in downtown Minneapolis, abandoning him there as a joke. When he told me about it later, he described how badly it hurt and scared him at a time when he was already feeling isolated.

Although I know he had incidents with friends that upset him, I also now know that it's not uncommon for young people grappling with psychosis to believe they have faced trauma that never actually occurred. Randy Michael had never previously discussed experiencing any trauma in his childhood. I believe that his psychosis was at the root of what he was feeling. Regardless, at the time, my heart ached for his anguish.

Despite our attempts to offer love, support, and care, his anger seemed to grow, and he began to send more distressing texts, inundating us with abusive, offensive, dark, and deeply hurtful messages and photos. Sometimes he threatened self-harm. But he also shared music he admired, including one piece he claimed had saved his life. All the music he shared was made by artists who glorified weed in their music and lifestyle. Tragically, some of these artists met untimely deaths due to gang violence or overdosing.

We offered to come visit him, concerned that he was living alone and not working outside of his house, but he turned us down. "No. I want to focus on my music and recording," he said. "It is going to take me a few months. I think I will be done by the end of June."

> ### You Need to Know
>
> Isolation has been shown to be connected to higher levels of marijuana use. Individuals who were self-isolated during the COVID-19 pandemic shutdowns were found to use 20 percent more cannabis than those who did not self-isolate.[62] Many youths who use substances will either use it with friends to feel calmer, to sleep better, or to escape. Up to 50 percent of adolescents who have used in the past thirty days use alone and in isolation.[63] One prevention strategy is to talk to youth about the risk of using in isolation and why it's best to avoid using marijuana as an escape; it's merely a temporary solution for a deeper, ongoing issue that needs to be worked through utilizing counseling, self-care (e.g., meditation), or both.

Paranoid and Panicked

As we were climbing into bed late on Sunday, March 14, Randy and I were startled by a phone call from an unfamiliar number. I picked up warily.

"Hello?"

"Mom! Dad! You must come and help me," replied our panicked and out-of-breath son. "The mob is after me! Uncle —— is part of the mob; they are going to kill Kevin and Nadia's baby. They are after me and they are coming to the house for you guys!"

Then he hung up. My heart was pounding against my chest,

---

[62] S. J. Bartel et al., "Self-Isolation: A Significant Contributor to Cannabis Use during the COVID-19 Pandemic," *Substance Abuse* 41, no. 4 (2020): 409–12, https://doi.org/10.1080/08897077.2020.1823550.

[63] S. Connolly et al., "Characteristics of Alcohol, Marijuana, and Other Drug Use among Persons Aged 13–18 Years Being Assessed for Substance Use Disorder Treatment—United States, 2014–2022," *Morbidity and Mortality Weekly Report* 73, no. 5 (2024): 93–98, https://doi.org/10.15585/mmwr.mm7305a1.

and my hands and body began to shake in fear. What in the world was going on?

We desperately tried to reach back out to Randy Michael, but every call went unanswered. Unable to sleep, we made calls to him throughout the night. By morning, we were deeply concerned. Seeking guidance, I contacted one of my brothers, who suggested arranging a "wellness check"—asking local police to stop by to check on him.

The police knocked on his apartment door that Monday afternoon. The officer noted that Randy Michael looked disheveled when he answered the door, but he reassured them that he was fine, "just indulging in a bit of weed."

The officer who had talked to our son called me to let me know he was okay, and he shared that he had a similar experience with his daughter. He told me that sometimes, regrettably, individuals need to get to their lowest point before getting help. This kind but disheartening insight felt like a foreshadowing of what lay ahead, and unfortunately, wellness checks would become routine for us over the next few months.

When Randy Michael called me that evening, his voice was again frantic and filled with distress. He said a blizzard had swept through Denver over the weekend and the "Taylor Gang" was hunting him down because of something he had posted online. He was convinced they were on their way to kill him.

He also told me he had been trapped in a freezing car during the storm and had contemplated slitting his wrists as an escape from the bitter cold. On top of that, he said he had attempted to break into several cars and was swept up into an ordeal that involved the police, but they inexplicably had let him go. He claimed there was tangible evidence of self-harm on his wrists, but he assured me he had halted because he didn't want to cause us any pain. Then he dropped an even more alarming revelation: he claimed to have taken drugs laced with meth from a dealer.

To this day, we are not sure exactly what happened that evening. We know a gang wasn't after him, and there was no record of any interaction with the police. He wasn't arrested, and I am certain he would have been detained if he had broken into cars. But he had been out running barefoot in a blizzard because his feet were frostbitten. And he tried to slit his wrists because he sent us photos of his sliced-up wrists, which were documented at Denver Health. His car was also impounded as it was found abandoned on the side of the road. We thought he was confused and severely depressed at this time, but we now know that he was having a full-blown psychotic event.

After two nights of panicked phone calls, I was reeling with disbelief and anxiety. Somehow, we managed to maintain composure, urging him to seek detox and possibly even treatment. To my astonishment, he agreed to both during our discussion—a glimmer of hope amid the chaos! It seemed like a breakthrough, a realization that his mental state was out of control; he needed urgent help. Grateful yet apprehensive, I whispered a prayer of thanks, hoping desperately that this might be the turning point we had been waiting for.

We reached out to a family friend named Greta. Greta had been one of Brooke's closest friends since childhood and is the sister to Alec, one of Randy Michael's childhood best friends. Greta was living in Denver, pursuing her master's degree in social work, and specializing in addiction. Greta had known Randy Michael since preschool, and she cared for him like a brother, so she headed to Randy Michael's apartment at about ten-thirty that Monday night to help us out.

Greta called me while taking Randy Michael to Denver Health Hospital for detox, and I remained on the line as he was admitted. Eventually, they transferred him to the emergency department concerned about his frostbitten feet and wheezing. The emergency department conducted an extensive battery of tests including CT scans, lung X-rays, and a five-panel drug test. They also administered acetaminophen and provided a Tdap vaccination.

As they waited for the doctor, Greta noticed Randy Michael was hearing nonexistent music. Following the medical assessments, Denver Health listed the reasons for his visit as a laceration, paranoia, and a substance use disorder with a severe dependence on cannabis. The five-panel drug test did not include THC, and remarkably enough, all that was detected in his system was amphetamine. His delirium still raised questions about what he had taken though, and Randy Michael kept insisting that had smoked something laced with something else. We were aware of his consistent marijuana use and knew he sometimes used other people's prescriptions of Adderall or Vyvanse. Maybe he had landed in the hospital because he had taken someone else's prescription medicine or what he thought was a prescription but was instead laced with amphetamines. It's also possible he smoked marijuana laced with meth. Unfortunately, we will never know.

Astonishingly, after a barrage of procedures, tests, and diagnoses, the hospital discharged him back to the streets by 6 a.m. on Tuesday. Greta had gone home after Randy Michael had been admitted, so there he was, all alone in a state of psychosis when he was discharged to the streets.

> ### *You Need to Know*
>
> Despite our plea for Randy Michael to receive detox care, he was discharged onto the streets without any form of ongoing support or guidance. Though he was clearly in a state of paranoia and psychosis, and experiencing auditory hallucinations, there was no provision of transportation or connection with a social worker to oversee his well-being. Shouldn't his mental instability have warranted hospitalization and follow-up care? He was paranoid with frostbitten feet due to running from a supposed gang, he had lacerations from trying to slit his wrists, and he was hearing music that wasn't in fact playing. How can a young person in that state of extreme distress and psychosis be discharged without detox care or at least a psychological evaluation? Sure, a severe dependence on cannabis was noted in his chart, but it seems no one understood what that actually meant for our son. It's distressing to acknowledge that our social and healthcare systems, which had failed Randy Michael during his high school years, continue to lack the necessary provisions for those struggling with mental health issues. This failure is particularly notable since the COVID-19 pandemic in which many individuals have been facing challenges with their mental well-being.[64]

Randy Michael phoned me after he was released from the emergency department, and I urged him to go back to detox. He said they had no available beds, but I checked and found out otherwise. He regretfully returned to the detox facility but chose not to stay when they attempted to take his phone. He insisted the phone was essential for his website work that he wanted to complete.

---

64 Ryan L. McBain, Jonathan H. Cantor, and Nicole K. Eberhart, "Estimating Psychiatric Bed Shortages in the US," *JAMA Psychiatry* 79, no. 4 (2022): 279, https://doi.org/10.1001/jamapsychiatry.2021.4462.

Randy Michael was markedly different from his usual self at this point. He seemed so malleable. Very childlike and flexible. I told him his dad was driving to Denver and would arrive by the end of the day and that I would be available by phone any time.

He requested an Uber to his apartment, and I stayed on the line until he safely arrived. He mentioned severe discomfort in his feet, likely due to the frostbite. He was exhausted, so I suggested he take a nap and call me when he woke. He phoned about forty-five minutes later, stating he was hungry, so I ordered him a pizza. I set my watch alarm as a reminder to contact him every forty-five minutes until his father arrived that evening. For the first time in so many nights, I was able to sleep knowing he was not alone, and his dad was there.

CHAPTER 10

DESPERATE LOVE

Cycling from Fear to Hope and Back Again

Before my husband, Randy, departed for Denver, we hugged goodbye and discussed how much patience he would need when dealing with our son. We knew that he would have to try to remain calm regardless of what happened. We also agreed not to push Randy Michael into treatment unless he voluntarily requested it. The wilderness therapy experience had made us wary of forcing Randy Michael into any sort of treatment.

When Randy arrived in Denver on Tuesday, March 16, he discovered that Randy Michael still feared he was being pursued by the mob and the Taylor Gang, was convinced his phone and computer were hacked, and felt an urgent need to contact the FBI. We tried our best to reassure him and redirect his thoughts, unaware that his delusions indicated a state of psychosis that could develop into a long-term condition, including schizophrenia or bipolar disorder.[65] We were likely in denial and perhaps a bit naive. As I have mentioned, in hindsight, it's clear how strong denial can be.

---

65 T. Schoeler, J. Ferris, and A. R. Winstock, "Rates and Correlates of Cannabis-Associated Psychotic Symptoms in Over 230,000 People Who Use Cannabis," *Translational Psychiatry* 12 (2022), https://doi.org/10.1038/s41398-022-02112-8.

Randy arrived at our son's apartment only to find it was littered with dirty dishes, blunts, and ash-filled bowls; it reeked of marijuana. They spent the next day cleaning the apartment and also discussed getting help for his addiction. Randy Michael initially agreed that he needed help, but after time with his dad, he suddenly switched his position on the matter and began to refuse all suggestions and thoughts about treatment.

Exhausted and growing more and more frustrated with the situation, Randy took a break, returning to his nearby hotel room for a nap. They agreed Randy Michael would drive the mile and a half to his dad's hotel later to pick him up so they could have dinner together.

But he called about the time they were supposed to meet, confused and disoriented. "Dad, I can't find you. How do I get to the restaurant?"

As soon as his dad had left the apartment, Randy Michael had reached for his marijuana, and he quickly became panicked and more paranoid.

"People are following me," he said. "They are coming to get me."

Randy reassured our son that he was safe. When they eventually got together, Randy Michael agreed once again that he needed help and wanted treatment.

Meanwhile, back at home, I was desperately searching for a suitable dual-diagnosis treatment center. A dual-diagnosis treatment center not only addresses addiction but co-occurring mental health issues as well. Often the two occur hand in hand.[66] I explored various programs, sought professional guidance, and

---

[66] National Institute on Drug Abuse, "The Connection between Substance Use Disorders and Mental Illness," April 2020, https://nida.nih.gov/publications/research-reports/common-comorbidities-substance-use-disorders/part-1-connection-between-substance-use-disorders-mental-illness.

discovered a ninety-day dual-diagnosis program in Boca Raton, Florida. At that time, the price tag for a private-pay situation was around seventy-five thousand dollars for a three-month stay, but that seemed preferable to Minnesota programs that were around fifty thousand dollars for thirty days without insurance.

We detailed Randy Michael's situation to the care team at the Florida treatment center, they conducted an interview with him over the phone, then agreed to admit him. They arranged for the on-staff psychiatrist to meet Randy Michael when he arrived but said he would first have to spend four days in a detox facility near the treatment center due to COVID restrictions.

Randy and Randy Michael flew to Fort Lauderdale on Friday, March 19. Randy Michael was picked up by staff from the detox center where he would begin his treatment and what we hoped would be his journey to recovery. We were so ignorant to believe it could be so simple.

Randy then returned to Denver with Randy Michael's cell phone and SIM card. Our goal was to handle our son's bills and other issues to ensure he could enter treatment without any concerns hanging over him. He took Randy Michael's damaged Nissan Leaf to the autobody shop, placed his Corvette in storage at a friend's place, and cleaned out his soiled apartment.

We expected Randy Michael would spend three months in the Florida treatment center, then move to a sober house or return home to Minnesota when he was released. Randy did not terminate Randy Michael's lease, but he discarded his mattress and desk chair, packed up his kitchen, dismantled his desk, and loaded his clothes and remaining belongings into our car. The entire apartment was now empty of his belongings.

Traveling overnight, Randy arrived home on Sunday, March 21. We were both emotionally drained, but also so relieved. Our son was finally going to receive the help he needed. He was in hands that knew how to deal with the agony he was experiencing in a way we could not. The detox center told us Randy Michael was stable and scheduled his transfer to the treatment center for Tuesday, March 23.

Reality Intrudes

Randy Michael was transferred to the treatment center on Tuesday, but after a single group therapy session, he urgently requested a FaceTime conversation with us. His therapist contacted us, concerned that Randy Michael was highly agitated and wanted to leave the program. The treatment center professionals advised us to try to force Randy Michael to stay by telling him we couldn't offer financial support, assist in his return home, or maintain communication if he left the program. Desperate, we followed their advice and prayed he would listen.

When we connected with Randy Michael via FaceTime around 10 a.m., he presented a detailed plan for achieving sobriety on his own. Despite his sincere intentions, we knew he could not handle this process alone. Although we were not fully aware, his severe addiction was compounded by hallucinations, delusions, and manic behavior. He adamantly insisted he could keep using marijuana. The treatment center staff warned us about potentially irreversible brain damage from his continued use. We wondered if the damage had already occurred.

No professional had explicitly labeled Randy Michael's issues as "cannabis-induced psychosis" or even said he had psychosis. Although we acknowledged his alarming behavior, we initially perceived it as a mood disorder rather than a drug-induced condition or mental illness. We had no idea that marijuana could cause psychosis that could lead to permanent schizophrenia or bipolar disorder, especially in young men ages sixteen to twenty-five.[67, 68]

In a fit of rage, Randy Michael abruptly left the treatment center, departing the campus without any possessions. He had no phone, credit cards, or money.

> ### *Hindsight*
>
> We were so relieved and happy to deliver Randy Michael to a facility that could help him fight his addiction. We anticipated that he had hit his rock bottom, and leaving treatment was never an option, but he wasn't in his right mind. We might have been more realistic if we had been more aware of the severity of Randy Michael's illness. I know now that we should have been prepared to take other actions, such as enforcing treatment via the Marchman Act, which allows for involuntary commitment in the state of Florida. The Marchman Act started in Florida in 1993. It provides a pathway to have persons with a substance use disorder involuntarily committed for evaluation, stabilization, and treatment under specific circumstances. The intention is to help those who are struggling and may not be in the best state of mind to make sound decisions. We so wish we would have known about this policy in March 2021. I often question, why didn't the treatment center in Florida know about it and recommend we utilize it?

---

67 A. Gonzalez-Pinto, S. Alberich, S. Barbeito, M. Gutierrez, P. Vega, B. Ibanez, M. K. Haidar, E. Vieta, and C. Arango, "Cannabis and First-Episode Psychosis: Different Long-Term Outcomes Depending on Continued or Discontinued Use." *Schizophrenia Bulletin* 37, no. 3 (2009): 631–39, https://doi.org/10.1093/schbul/sbp126.

68 Tabea Schoeler, Anna Monk, Musa B. Sami, Ewa Klamerus, Enrico Foglia, Ruth Brown, Giulia Camuri, A. Carlo Altamura, Robin Murray, and Sagnik Bhattacharyya, "Continued versus Discontinued Cannabis Use in Patients with Psychosis: A Systematic Review and Meta-Analysis," *The Lancet Psychiatry* 3, no. 3 (2016): 215–25, https://doi.org/10.1016/s2215-0366(15)00363-6.

Again, we found ourselves on an emotional roller coaster. Our twenty-one-year-old son, grappling with addiction and struggling to function, had walked out of the treatment center we had worked so hard to get him into. Now he was in southern Florida with no place to stay, no access to money, and no clear plan on how he would get back to Colorado. We were in Minnesota, grappling with frustration, disappointment, worry, uncertainty, and profound sadness. Treatment center staff kept telling us to hold firm to our boundaries and suggested how we might track Randy Michael if he reached out. They encouraged us to have him return to the center to retrieve his belongings so that they could attempt to persuade him to stay once again.

Hours later, a surprisingly calm Randy Michael called us and firmly declared his intention to return to Colorado to resume his website business, record his music, develop his clothing line—and continue his marijuana use.

We urged him to revisit the treatment center to gather his belongings, which he eventually did. He told his therapist there that he had hitchhiked to Boca with someone who had marijuana and smoked with her. The therapist noted that Randy Michael was more composed and sensible than he had been since arriving at the facility. No surprise: he had gotten his marijuana fix.

After gathering his belongings, Randy Michael contacted us from the phone store and bank, pleading for financial assistance. We refused and begged him to return to the treatment facility. Instead, he declared he was headed to Miami.

He called multiple times, desperately seeking our help to return to Colorado.

We repeatedly said no.

He reached out to others, including Aaron's mom and his childhood best friend, Alec, both caring individuals who had always tried to guide him. Alec, with immense maturity and compassion, gently said, "I can't in good conscience send you money. I believe you're right where you need to be." In taking that difficult path, Alec showed his genuine love, care, and concern for his friend and acted in his best interest.

While spending the next four nights in a Miami hotel, Randy Michael reached out repeatedly to threaten self-harm. He told us he was planning to jump off a building or do a "speedball," which we Googled and learned was taking a deadly combination of lethal drugs. We were on edge, and each time he made a threat, we contacted the Miami police for a wellness check. When authorities located him, Randy Michael claimed he was "okay" and dismissed the situation as a "family rift."

While playing nice with the police, Randy Michael was directing intense anger toward his dad, sending distressing messages and unsettling images to all of us.

You Need to Know

If your loved one is making threatening statements about harming themselves or others, keep a log, because a record of such threats can help you take legal action to get them help. It is possible in most states to commit your loved one to a facility to get help. We didn't know this until after we lost Randy Michael. Ask for help to determine what steps you need to take in your location to have a loved one committed involuntarily. In Florida, you can commit someone using the previously mentioned Marchman Act or by way of the Baker Act—officially the Florida Mental Health Act of 1971. It is for people showing evidence of mental illness and who are in danger of harming themselves or others.

Back Where We Started

On Saturday, March 28, Randy Michael used his credit card to purchase a plane ticket back to Colorado. He messaged us that he was on a flight back to Denver. Although I was devastated that he wasn't receiving treatment, I was relieved when he landed in Denver. At least he had shelter there.

But Randy Michael was furious when he returned to his barren apartment. We had cleared it out and taken his possessions to Minnesota, not anticipating his return there so soon. Randy Michael had only what fit in his suitcase for the trip to Florida, and he began demanding that we transport all his belongings back to Colorado.

Initially, we said, "No." Yet after a series of contentious exchanges marked by more disrespect, threats, and anger, we ultimately decided to FedEx everything back to him and draw a line.

Before shipping the boxes, we opened each one and took a photograph so he could not accuse us of keeping any of his items. The only items we did not ship back were his snow skis, boots, and a box of ammunition. The ski season was just about over, and he didn't have a gun, so he didn't need any ammunition.

Of course, once he received the boxes, he accused us of keeping some of his items. He was especially agitated over a food saver, several hundred plastic baggies, and a package of mailing labels. His agitation confirmed what we suspected—he was using those items to sell and distribute drugs by mail. After going through all the boxes we shipped to him, he eventually found his supplies, and we think he was relieved. He could be back in business as a "plug"—today's term for a drug dealer.

You Need to Know

Teens can often acquire a medical marijuana card for minor issues such as migraines or PTSD. This easy access can allow eighteen-year-olds to then sell to their younger friends or siblings.

As of January 2024, there were 65,620 registered medical marijuana participants in the Colorado program, including 57 who were ages ten or younger and 96 who were ages eleven to seventeen. However, registrations increased by more than tenfold to 1,013 participants who were eighteen to twenty.

Our son obtained his medical marijuana card in 2019, before the enactment of a law that significantly tightened up medical marijuana regulations in Colorado. At that time, the number of medical marijuana cardholders jumped from 162 in the eleven-to-seventeen age bracket to 3,362 for eighteen- to twenty-year-olds.

    Once we shipped Randy Michael's belongings to him, we told him we would not be in touch anymore. However, we notified him that we had inserted his old SIM card into an extra phone at home and that he could reach out to us using his old phone number when he felt ready to get help. We kept the "bat phone," as I referred to it, on our nightstands, checking it every morning, afternoon, and evening hoping that maybe, just maybe, Randy Michael would say he was ready to get help. Unfortunately, he was too sick to make rational decisions.

    Randy Michael utilized the bat phone regularly and often—but not to ask for help. Instead, he called to berate us and make more threats about his life, leading us to request more wellness checks. Eventually, he started threatening to come to our house and harm his dad. One day he sent a photo of what appeared to be a newly purchased gun. With a pit in my stomach, I sought professional guidance and was advised to block contact with him completely. Finally, the whole family did, although it was heartbreaking to do so.

Promises and Threats and Frustrations

In early April, Randy Michael reached out via the bat phone to suggest we do family therapy, convinced it would fix everything. We talked to professionals at the treatment center who said family therapy could be a starting point, a way to engage with Randy Michael on his terms—aligning with the Substance Abuse and Mental Health Services Administration's concept of meeting people where they are at.

On Easter Sunday, April 4, Randy Michael sent me a photo of the program from the Church of the Good Shepherd Parish in Cherry Creek, saying he "enjoyed Mass" and was planning to make regular attendance a part of his routine. Then he mentioned finding a therapist named "Jenny" who was willing to engage in family therapy. He begged me to contact her, and I assured him I would reach out the following day. I was grateful he went to church and genuinely surprised that a therapist responded on Easter, attributing it all to God's goodness.

I spoke with Jenny the next day and shared Randy Michael's background with her. She described her experience working with individuals dealing with marijuana addiction, including her son who had struggled with it for nearly ten years. She also told me she had connections to psychiatrists and would insist Randy Michael schedule an evaluation at the psychiatry office.

On April 6, Randy Michael sent us both a text and video message that he was willing to go to treatment. In the video, he rubs his eyes with a surgical mask under his chin, sighs, and states, "I'd really like to get help while I still have my brain." Elated, I immediately reached out to the treatment facility in Florida, which agreed to accept him back. But when I dialed Randy Michael to share the good news, he abruptly changed his mind, dismissing the idea entirely. He claimed he had discovered a YouTube channel that could assist him with his addiction and believed he could then aid others as well.

He again mentioned that he suspected his former roommate had been lacing his drugs, which triggered the psychotic episode. Then he said he intended to purchase a gun for self-protection.

As soon as our conversation ended, I searched for the State of Colorado firearms laws and regulations, even calling the Colorado Department of Public Health and Environment to better understand the process of obtaining a gun. To my surprise, having an arrest record was the only obstacle to acquiring one. Randy Michael had no criminal history, and within forty-eight hours, he was proudly sharing images of his brand-new Glock pistol.

Concerned friends alerted us to social media postings of his newly purchased gun, and not long after, Randy Michael began sending these images to us as a type of threat directed at his father. It again felt like our son had reached a breaking point, and I fervently prayed that he would remain safe and not pose a threat to anyone.

I informed Jenny, his therapist, that he now owned a firearm and had been making threats against his father. She then insisted that Randy Michael consult with the psychiatrist before his scheduled appointment with her. Surprisingly, he cooperated and scheduled an appointment at the psychiatry office.

On Sunday, April 18, I was awakened by a 7 a.m. call.

"Hello? Mrs. Bacchus? This is Dr. M from Denver Health. Your son, Randy, checked in because he was suicidal last night. He called the police, and they came to his apartment. He had a gun and said he was going to hurt himself. The police confiscated the gun. Has your son threatened to commit suicide in the past week?"

I answered, "Yes, several times."

The doctor asked a few more questions and then stated, "Okay, I am going to put him on an involuntary seventy-two-hour hold and have him committed."

Finally! Thank you, God! We were elated and hopeful once again!

However, that afternoon, the bat phone started ringing. It was Randy Michael.

"Mom, I'm okay. I want to go home. I have job interviews this week. Last night, I did some mushrooms, and they set my mind right. I feel much better. Can you please talk to the doctor and tell them to let me go?"

"You need to discuss this with your doctor," I replied. "He's the expert."

Randy Michael called again a few hours later. "Mom, I feel so much better. I'm so sorry for all the horrible things I said to you and especially to Dad."

His voice sounded like the son we once knew, but I replied, "I'm sorry, Randy, but I think you're in the right place. The doctor will make the right decision."

Around 10:30 that night, the doctor phoned me. "Mrs. Bacchus, this is Dr. M. . . . Your son Randy is here and wants to leave. There are no available beds, and since he's no longer a threat to himself or others, we're releasing him. Even if there were beds, since he is no longer suicidal, they would let him go. You know your son. He's young, and you have a long road ahead."

Those were his exact words. Little did we know, our "long" road would come to a literal dead end.

He added, "You could have Randy undergo court-ordered treatment, but Colorado lacks lockdown facilities, allowing him to walk off campus if he wanted to. It's impossible to force someone to stay in treatment once they're eighteen, even when they're very ill."

Sadly, Randy Michael was discharged shortly after our conversation.

There was no mention of cannabis-induced psychosis—or any diagnosis at all. The doctor simply acknowledged our son was difficult to work with and suffered from addiction. I am disappointed in the care our son received in a state that has recorded increased incidences of cannabis-induced psychosis, cannabis hyperemesis syndrome, and cannabis poisonings since marijuana use was legalized. The doctors knew Randy Michael's level of use; they should have looked at his chart history noting a substance use disorder, a previous suicide attempt, and hospitalization. If the doctor cared, shouldn't he have told us our son was suffering a mental health crisis caused or exacerbated by drug use and given us a diagnosis?

> ## *Hindsight*
>
> Because no healthcare professional ever diagnosed Randy Michael with anything beyond a substance use disorder, we often assumed he was developmentally healthy but difficult. We didn't realize that marijuana could arrest development and disrupt homeostasis in the developing brain, leading to mental health issues, including suicidal ideation. If Randy Michael had received a diagnosis indicating that cannabis was contributing to or was the root cause of his mental health issues, we would have better understood his difficult personality. We could have dissociated his behavior from his person and been less afraid of him as an individual.

CHAPTER 11

PERSISTENT LOVE

Pursuing Healing, Stability

Randy Michael insisted he needed to leave the lockdown facility because he had job interviews. I knew he was telling the truth about the interviews because we had access to his email account and knew he had been applying for jobs and attending multiple interviews. Right after returning from Florida, he had managed to get positions as a pizza delivery driver and a marijuana shop tour guide, but neither job had lasted long. Just two days after he was hospitalized, Randy Michael successfully interviewed for a property management job that was set to start at the beginning of May.

Facing financial strain, he eagerly looked forward to resuming full-time work and remained optimistic, determined to regain stability.

When we refused to loan him money, Randy Michael accepted our decision without displaying any anger or frustration, which was unusual for him in the past six months. Although we refused to directly support him because we did not want to enable his continued marijuana use, we certainly did not want to see our son homeless or hungry, so I suggested he seek emergency assistance from the parish he had started attending.

We saw through his email account that he followed through, and the church graciously provided financial support for his rent and food for two months. We felt blessed by the generosity extended to him during a challenging time.

Despite his internal and external chaos, Randy Michael remained incredibly diligent about managing his finances. Before he departed for Colorado years prior, I gave him a book titled *Why Didn't They Teach Me This in School?* by Cary Siegel, which covered a wide array of topics, including finances. When we sorted through his belongings after his passing, we discovered Randy Michael had marked every single page in the financial section with a sticky note, which made me immensely proud of his commitment to educating himself, yet profoundly sad to know how much he struggled in his final months. He was still trying to keep ahead of his bills even as he became more conscious of his cognitive struggles.

In late April, Randy Michael finally underwent an evaluation at the psychiatry clinic and began in-person sessions with Jenny. We agreed to cover all of Randy Michael's appointment expenses if he would share pertinent information with us and let us communicate with his providers—something he readily agreed to. Jenny was committed to guiding Randy Michael, regularly updating us on their discussions and his progress.

I was anxiously anticipating the diagnosis from the psychiatrist when I contracted a bad case of COVID-19 in early May. It hit me hard, limiting my communication with Randy Michael for nearly two weeks. He periodically checked in through the bat phone with brief texts, telling us he was enjoying the new job and diving deeper into music recording and his web design business. He also softened and sent his dad this email on May 6, 2021:

May 6, 2021

Hey Dad,

I know that I said a lot of things. I had a lot of anger from whatever I was taking. Something switched and didn't switch back till I went to the hospital. I miss you and am sorry that I have been such a disappointment. At this point I am taking ownership of the mess that I got myself into. I was childish, out of line, and now have to pay for my mistakes.

I appreciate you trying to help me. I am sorry for everything I said. Truly. I have been going to mass again and have been trying to put my future in a better position. As I think I got lost. . . .

I think that things that frustrated me about our past and paranoia from the laced drugs that I got put me in a really dark place and thankfully I am out of that place. Don't plan on going back.

I hope that one day we can patch things up and was very happy to hear that you were going to be coming to family therapy. I had to refamiliarize myself with the 10 commandments and I was not honoring you. At all.

I did not mean to have things get this out of control and am blessed that you came all the way out to help. I was paranoid when you came out and didn't think that you really loved me because you were so tense. I also had all of this anger from my past resurface.

I am excited to be starting a real estate/leasing position with a cool company and to be feeling like myself again. I have created a plan for how I am going to get my life together. Just to let you know what I have been up to.

I love you and hope we get to have a meaningful future at some point. I love you and am sorry for everything that I said. It was really mean and disrespectful to everything that you have done.

I know that you tried your best. I am blessed to have had you in my life for as long as I have. You have already lost enough and I am sorry if I have ruined things forever.

I hope you have a good day and that we can see each other in the near future. I do love you Dad. I hope you are doing well.

Love,
Your son Randy —
Randy Bacchus III

On May 9, the nurse practitioner from the psychiatrist's office reached out to discuss Randy Michael's recent diagnosis, which included

- Psychosis (resolved)
- Bipolar disorder
- ADHD
- PTSD
- Mood disorder
- Anxiety
- Depression

This list overwhelmed us and convinced us that Randy Michael needed much more care than he was getting, but he was adamant that he would heal on his own. The nurse practitioner noted that Randy Michael was reluctant to take any medication aside from Adderall for his ADHD and he was quite clear that he intended to continue using marijuana. She strongly advised against continued use and demanded a clean drug test before she would prescribe Adderall for his ADHD. However, I don't know if she explained why marijuana use was so bad for Randy Michael.

In mid-May, Randy Michael landed a second job washing windows and buildings in Denver. This side gig paid in cash and allowed him to work in the evenings after his property management job had ended. The hours often stretched past midnight and encroached into his weekends, but Randy Michael expressed genuine satisfaction with the job, praising the company owner. However, he would frequently text us in the dead of night or the early morning hours, so I knew he was getting little to no sleep, which concerned me.

You Need to Know

Marijuana can disrupt sleep schedules, especially with acute or chronic use.[69] Marijuana may also trigger manic behavior.[70]

The Concern and Love from Friends

By May 23, Randy Michael appeared more levelheaded, so we agreed to accept his calls and emails on our phones with the

---

[69] Gustavo A. Angarita et al., "Sleep Abnormalities Associated with Alcohol, Cannabis, Cocaine, and Opiate Use: A Comprehensive Review," *Addiction Science & Clinical Practice* 11, no. 1 (April 2016), https://doi.org/10.1186/s13722-016-0056-7.

[70] Melanie Gibbs et al., "Cannabis Use and Mania Symptoms: A Systematic Review and Meta-analysis," *Journal of Affective Disorders* 171 (2015): 39–47, https://doi.org/10.1016/j.jad.2014.09.016.

caveat that his communication remain respectful and nonthreatening. He seemed to be doing well through the first weeks of June even while juggling two jobs, dedicating time to recording music, and maintaining his cannabis use.

On June 10, he crossed paths with Greta and Alec's dad, who had come to Denver to celebrate Greta's graduation from her master's program. The family had organized a pizza party and invited Randy Michael over to join them. Randy Michael told Alec and Greta that he had taken an edible before he arrived. Initially he seemed to enjoy the gathering, but suddenly his demeanor shifted, and he became paranoid and departed abruptly.

I am sure the encounter with his friend's family was complex for Randy Michael. I messaged Randy Michael after seeing photos of him with the family. He called me and said, "It was good to see them, but they were talking shit about me behind my back, and I had to leave."

I knew that this family cherished Randy Michael deeply and I tried to persuade him that no one had been talking negatively about him. His belief persisted, and the sorrow in his voice during that conversation broke my heart. It was so distressing to hear my son feeling persecuted by people who truly loved him and had his best interests in mind. Now I realize that the sorrow in Randy Michael's voice was actually his hope slowly fading away and voices of deceit taking over his mind.

On June 12, a couple of days after Randy Michael's encounter with our family friends, another one of his childhood friends, "Nina," reached out to me. She had been involved in modeling for Randy Michael's clothing line in January 2021, but his behavior and repeated hurtful remarks prompted Nina's younger brothers to demand that he end all contact with her. Randy Michael distanced himself from her then, but he chose to call her early on June 12 to wish her a Happy Birthday. Following their conversation, Nina then reached out to me, as Randy Michael was extremely intoxicated during the call; she was worried and concerned, and rightfully so.

Although we had not spoken since the incident in which Randy Michael had been so rude to her, Nina and I candidly discussed Randy Michael's situation and their recent negative interactions. I confided in her about his struggle with addiction and how he refused our repeated offers of help, insisting that he could navigate sobriety independently. Remember, at this time, I was unaware he was in and out of a psychotic state.

To this day, I have the utmost respect for Nina for her mature, brave, and compassionate phone call. She genuinely cared for Randy Michael's well-being and epitomized a true friend who was invested in his welfare. Only a few of Randy Michael's friends and acquaintances were ever courageous enough to reach out to us and express their concern for our son, and we are deeply grateful for the presence of those genuine friends in his life. Their care and bravery in stepping forward was incredibly valuable.

Nina's phone call and other small signs continued to feed our growing concern for Randy Michael, even though in some ways he seemed to be stabilizing. To help provide the whole picture to his therapist, I continued to reach out to Jenny, sharing details I suspected he might not have disclosed.

Around June 18, Randy Michael called me and said, "Hey, Mom, I've started taking Adderall, so I don't feel the need to smoke as much. But I'll continue until I finish my album."

He was sure that he would soon become a prominent rap artist and achieve wealth and fame with his music and clothing line. He was also sure that he needed to continue using marijuana to enhance his creativity and facilitate the completion of his music. We reiterated our concerns about his aspirations, expressed doubts about Adderall being sufficient medication for the multiple issues noted by the psychiatrist, and stressed the importance of following his doctor's advice to stop using marijuana. He claimed he had told the psychiatrist he had stopped using weed, but then told us that he planned to continue using it. Once more we urged Randy Michael to heed the doctor's suggestion, which again triggered his anger.

> ### You Need to Know
>
> Thoroughly vet all care providers. Take time to interview them, find out their credentials, and do your due diligence. If a loved one is put on medication, conduct your own research, and ask specific questions with the prescriber. Become familiar with how medications work, what illnesses are its primary indications, and possible side effects. Adderall, for example, is not an FDA-approved medication for bipolar disorder.[71]

Glimmers of Stability, but a Mountain of Bills

In mid-June, Randy Michael received a fifteen-thousand-dollar hospital bill for his detox and Emergency Department stay in March, along with an additional seven-thousand-dollar tab for the twenty-four-hour mental health hold in April. He was distressed by the bill, and I could hear the anxiety in his voice when he called to tell me about it. I encouraged him to reach out to his Christian Health Share plan which is an alternative to traditional insurance and to the hospital to explore his coverage and payment options.

---

71 Kate Levenberg and Zachary A. Cordner, "Bipolar Depression: A Review of Treatment Options," *General Psychiatry* 35, no. 4 (August 2022), https://doi.org/10.1136/gpsych-2022-100760.

> ### *Hindsight*
>
> Because we were trying to hold him accountable for his actions, I expected Randy Michael to take care of his medical bills on his own and seek help when needed. Later, we learned that he was receiving persistent collection notices at his apartment when we gathered his mail after his passing. Although I offered ideas about steps he could take to pay off his bills, I wish now that I had set up three-way calls so I could advocate for him more directly. No one else was looking out for him in the hospital billing system. Three-way calls are simple and easy to do on a cell phone. I simply did not understand how damaged his brain was and did not realize I was asking too much of him in this case.

A week after Randy Michael received the hospital bills, Randy Michael, my husband, and I engaged in a family therapy session with Jenny via FaceTime. Randy Michael appeared in good spirits and at one point asked us, "Could you at least acknowledge how terrifying it was for me during the blizzard in March?"

> ### *Hindsight*
>
> We didn't quite understand Randy Michael's past trauma or how/why he was officially diagnosed with posttraumatic stress disorder (PTSD), and sometimes we were not as empathetic as we should have been. Looking back now, it is much easier to understand why and how he was fixated on his PTSD, continuing to seek out our understanding. He was often in a state of psychosis, paranoia, and/or delusion, uncertain of what was and was not real, so many things were likely triggers for him because he wasn't perceiving things correctly or processing things in his brain as he should have been.

During the remainder of the family therapy session with Jenny, we tried to empathetically acknowledge the fear he experienced, even though we still did not know exactly what had happened to him. I also gently urged him to recognize the inherent risk involved in consuming drugs, emphasizing they can often be laced with unknown substances including toxic chemicals, pesticides, and metals. I wish I had also shared how detrimental marijuana was to his developing brain and how it had impacted him, but we just didn't know that information or the extent of its destruction on his brain at the time.

Surprisingly, instead of reacting with anger, Randy Michael began to discuss his past choices. We eventually redirected the conversation, emphasizing the need to move forward, as we cannot change the past. We proposed setting achievable goals—looking ahead to a year, a month, a week, a day, and even an hour—and we urged him to focus on living in the present moment. He appeared receptive to our suggestions, and the session concluded with "I love you" sentiments from everyone. We all agreed it would be beneficial to continue online face-to-face meetings monthly. Randy and I felt cautiously hopeful.

From that date on, we maintained daily contact with Randy Michael through calls or texts, and he appeared to be in good spirits. During our conversations, he discussed his music recordings, his leasing agent career, and washing windows for extra income. He even expressed gratitude toward us, acknowledging his challenging behavior and recognizing that he had been blessed with a privileged, loving, supportive, and sheltered upbringing.

It warmed our hearts to witness him exhibit more stability, contentment, and appreciation, but our concern for his well-being lingered. From his emails, I could see his continuous job applications at odd hours of the night and frequent visits to the dispensary. We were acutely aware of the unpredictable nature of addiction, a constant roller coaster of highs and lows that we had been riding for years.

Desperately wanting to see him, we asked if we could visit him over the Fourth of July holiday, but he said no.

"I need to work on recording my album and get this thing knocked out," he said. "I'll be coming home at the end of August to release my album and promote it at the Minnesota State Fair."

His aspirations of musical success continued to make us uneasy, yet we refrained from expressing our reservations. While we doubted his chances of becoming a famous rapper, we remained uncertain about what the future held and worried that another crisis was coming.

On July 4, I sent Randy Michael a copy of a poem (see Figure 11.1) he had crafted when he was eleven years old—a precious relic from a happier time.

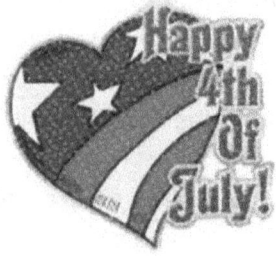

Happy 4th of July to every one...
And may every thing glow and sparkle your way.
Put all your spirit and joy to use.
Possess as many fireworks as possible.
You should remember those who gave us
independence.

Feel proud for your country.
Over excitement shall come your way.
Unite with others during this time.
Roman candles could be headed your way.
Therefore be careful, but still enjoy yourself.
Help others if your help is needed.

Over achieve at whatever you choose to do.
For today we celebrate how America achieved
freedom for us.

Jump in excitement for our country.
Use every bit of happiness that you have.
Let yourself enjoy the view.
Yet remember what America has done for us!

Figure 11.1. An early patriotic acrostic

He replied by saying he loved me and missed me.

Our oldest daughter, Brooke, was planning to visit friends in the Denver/Boulder area over the Fourth of July holiday, and she discussed with us whether she should meet up with Randy Michael. Our daughters had cut off communication with their brother in late March because of his threats and instability, and Brooke worried about seeing him, despite his apparent recent improvements in behavior. Known for her peacemaking nature, Brooke had always tried to mend situations for her brother both in his childhood and adolescence, but Randy Michael's manipulative actions and words had deeply affected his sisters. Witnessing how his behavior impacted us as a whole over the past five years also gave her reason to pause and question if a visit would be beneficial at this time.

After a morning hike with friends, Brooke decided to reach out to her brother and asked if he would meet for lunch in Boulder. It was July 5. During their time together, Brooke expressed concern for his mental and physical well-being, conveying her love and genuine desire for his happiness. She said he seemed despondent, fatigued, and thin, which was evident in the pictures she shared of their meeting. I am sure it was emotionally taxing for Randy Michael to reconnect with Brooke, as he repeated expressions of remorse and apologized to her during their visit. To me, this highlighted that he was aware of his behavior and maybe even how it impacted her and our family.

Given his conscientious disposition and longing for acceptance, it's likely he grappled with feelings of shame, guilt, sadness, and loneliness, compounded by psychotic symptoms because of his drug use.

Brooke told us she gave Randy Michael an extended, firm hug during their farewell.

When he asked, "Why did you do that?" she replied, "I needed to."

I'll forever cherish Brooke's tender decision to meet with Randy Michael. With love and care for her brother, she voiced her concern, offered an enduring embrace, and took in his radiant smile and striking face. Unbeknownst to Brooke, this would be their last visit together. The regret of not seeing him during those chaotic months weighs heavily on me nearly every single day. Would he still be here if I had insisted on seeing him?

That same day, Randy Michael reached out to us seeking prayers for his album's success and the possibility of a new job. I assured him of our prayers while gently reminding him of the music industry's challenges.

A few days later, he told me about a new job opportunity he was pursuing in the auto loan industry. He was excited because it was a remote job and that meant he could come back to Minnesota and stay with us more frequently.

We continued to communicate daily and were beginning to feel more confident that he was growing more stable. On July 13, he mentioned going to Confession and said it might "be a long one." Later, he told us with sincerity that the best thing about Confession was that he no longer had to say, "I'm sorry." It was as if a weight had been lifted off his shoulders. It seems he not only said it but genuinely believed it. As his mom, that makes my heart so happy.

Following his session with Jenny on July 15, he texted, "Session with Jenny went well!"

Knowing he was worried about his financial status, I texted him a link to an article on various ways of handling medical bills. He never responded to it.

CHAPTER 12

FORGIVING LOVE

I'm Sorry for Everything. . . . Me too. I love you.

When we talked with Randy Michael on Friday evening, July 16, he was sad and frustrated, dismayed that he had sent $600 to someone to mix his music and that he owed $2,100 for repairs to his Corvette. Our youngest daughter, Anna, Randy, and I had Randy Michael on speakerphone while we were watching TV from our bed. Our dog, Herbie, cuddled up beside us.

I wasn't exactly sure why Randy Michael was upset about the money he had spent on his music. I couldn't tell if he was dissatisfied with the outcome or just reconsidering the investment. But he thought the mechanic had caused the problem he was having with his Corvette and then demanded money to fix it.

He asked me for advice on small claims court, and I shared about my own fruitless pursuit against a moving company that had damaged our furniture in a move from Florida to Minnesota. I explained it was a process that could eat up time and energy without a guarantee of any kind of refund.

I said I didn't think small claims court was worth the effort but advised him to research the process for himself. We again cautioned him about potential exploitation within the music production business, and I was a little astonished that he seemed to be listening attentively instead of reacting negatively or getting angry.

We talked for about half an hour and were surprised when he called back around 9:30 p.m. It seemed like he simply called to say, "I love you."

I said, "I love you too. What are your plans for tomorrow?"

"I have to work tomorrow," he responded and kind of lingered.

"Well, we are going to watch a movie now," I said. "I love you and will talk with you tomorrow, okay?"

"I love you too," Randy Michael responded. "Good night."

How many times have I replayed that conversation in my head? How many times have I wished for another chance to give him better advice? How many times have I wanted to rewind our discussion and offer him more encouragement? To remind him that tomorrow will be a better day?

At 11:19 p.m., he texted me: "Have a good night. I love you and can't wait to get this stuff knocked out and settled next year."

He added, "Say hi to the girls, too," and added a heart emoji. I replied, "Will do. I love you too. Good night."

Overnight Messages, Then Silence

When I woke up on Saturday morning, I reached for my phone and read the text that had arrived from Randy Michael at 1:26 a.m.:

> My attitude with the music and everything has been way too self-righteous. I am done with the music. I'm quitting weed for good and want to surround myself with healthy

> and happy people. This has been too much for you guys. I have been running from my past mistakes, and it's time that I own up and start living a good life. Love you.

I had a moment of hopeful joy, but my heart dropped when I read his next message, which had arrived less than an hour later, at 2:09 a.m.:

> I love you and am sorry for everything. I love Dad, and the same to him. I wish I would have been a better person.

I had a fleeting sense that Randy Michael might be gone, but I brushed it aside and clung to the hope that this text was an "I love you" rather than a "goodbye."

About six hours after I had received Randy Michael's last text, I sent him a morning greeting:

> Good morning Randy. Thanks for the text. That sounds like a good plan. We hope you have a good day. Life isn't easy, things happen, and we all make choices. It is never too late to make changes and start something new. Today is a fresh start. We love you too.

What I did not know was that July 17, 2021, marked Randy Michael's fresh start in his heavenly life. And the beginning of our earthly hell.

Randy and I both sent individual texts to Randy Michael that morning and then tried reaching out in a group text. We did not receive any response. But since he had told us the night before that he would be working on Saturday, his silence did not initially worry us too much; we assumed he was occupied with work. When we did not hear back from him on Sunday, we assumed he was busy with his power-washing gig.

Although I was struggling with a sense of unease after reading his text Saturday morning, I believe our ability to rationalize his lack of response was the result of divine intervention. Brooke, who had made plans to fly home from Texas to escape the heat, arrived on Sunday evening. I believe God's timing ensured that she would be with us when we could no longer deny reality.

By Monday morning, anxiety gnawed at me. Randy Michael had not called or texted all weekend. We sent out another group text that went unanswered, and I began making other attempts to contact him. I tried to contact the leasing company where he worked and left a voicemail when no one answered the phone.

By 3:00 p.m., my mounting worry drove me to action, and I reached out to the Denver police, asking them to do a wellness check at our son's apartment.

Later that afternoon, Randy Michael's manager at the leasing office returned my call. She told me that Randy Michael had not shown up for work on Saturday and she had unsuccessfully attempted to contact him multiple times that day.

Annoyed, she stated, "Mondays are his day off, and I haven't seen him."

This new information only compounded our worries.

Around 4:30 p.m., a Denver police officer called and asked about Randy Michael's cars. We told him he owned two and described them. The officer said both vehicles were parked at his location.

The officer promised to follow up and left us waiting again. When we had previously asked for wellness checks, officers had swiftly contacted Randy Michael and then called to reassure us of his well-being. This lack of response felt ominous.

I had no appetite but made dinner for the girls.

At 6:30 p.m., I contacted the police department again. The

woman who answered indicated that the officer would have an update in about an hour.

My prayers intensified.

"Please, God, let him be okay. Don't let them find him."

My mind raced with unsettling scenarios: "Is he lost on the streets? Could he be hurt, wandering, or worse?"

I recited a Hail Mary, pleading for the Virgin Mary to interfere like I had so many other times, to watch over him in our absence.

Eventually, my prayer transitioned to, "God, let Your will be done."

The Call That Changed It All

Around 9:15 p.m., my husband, Randy, and I were working in our separate home offices upstairs when my phone rang, displaying a Colorado number. I put the caller on speakerphone.

"Hello, Mrs. Bacchus? This is [. . .] from the Denver County Coroner's office. We have your son, Randy Bacchus, here. He is deceased. It appears he died by suicide."

The words came in a rapid, staccato tone that jolted through me like an electric shock, leaving me shaking uncontrollably. I barely registered anything beyond "deceased."

Tearful, dizzy, and breathless, I pleaded, "Please, slow down. Can you please stop?"

The caller repeated that it seemed Randy Michael died by suicide, having shot himself. In a monotone voice, she mentioned a police investigation and assured us a detective would contact us soon.

The call ended, and Randy and I held each other, engulfed in tears. Our worst nightmare was now reality. Recalling that moment today still makes me feel as if I cannot breathe.

Our daughters knew, of course, about our concern for Randy Michael and that we had requested a wellness check. We met Brooke and Anna downstairs after the call, and they read the grief on our faces and instantly understood what it meant. We hugged, sobbed, and unsuccessfully sought comfort in each other's arms. A bit later, Sabrina returned home from a friend's and found us sitting in silence and disbelief. One of us broke the silence to tell her the news and tears streamed down her face as she collapsed into us and joined in our mourning.

Our hearts shattered into countless pieces, each one of us irreparably broken.

We went to bed without calling anyone else. Why would we steal from them the peace of one more night's sleep? There was nothing to be done until morning. On many worrisome nights, I often clutched the rosary to my chest, trying to find ease and rest. That night was no different, but sleep evaded me. Our girls slept three to a bed that night, woken up intermittently by the sobs of one another, and eventually in the morning to the sobs of two parents who realized that the nightmare they had the night before was reality.

CHAPTER 13
THE GRIEF OF LOVE

Picking Up the Pieces

When morning arrived, we began to reach out to others. One by one, we called close friends and family to tell them what had happened. Within minutes, our doorbell rang, and we were surrounded by love and support. We will forever be grateful for that outpouring.

We also reached out to our guiding beacon, Father Talbot. He prayed with and for us and for Randy Michael and our entire extended family. He also steered us toward a mortician who helped us handle the logistical challenges that arise when a loved one passes away out of state. Father Talbot recommended blessing Randy Michael's body before his cremation, which meant we had to decide whether to have his body embalmed for viewing. It felt surreal to have to make such choices for our son in general and so quickly.

The enormity of the decisions overwhelmed us. I had not seen our son in person since September 2020. Although many suggested viewing his body might benefit our family, I didn't necessarily want to see Randy Michael's face, but I had an inexplicable need to see his hands. I shared that feeling with Father Talbot, Randy, the mortician, and my sister.

Randy Michael possessed the most exquisite hands—even from birth. Shortly after he was born, my mom noted he had "big paws" and would probably make a fine piano player someday. As an adult, he had long, thin fingers with well-groomed nails. I kept thinking about raking the yard one fall day when Randy Michael was just a little guy. As we walked, he held my hand, looked up, and sang the song "You're Beautiful" by James Blunt. As he grew older, he would often hold my hand while we watched movies on the couch, my hand feeling smaller and smaller with each passing year.

After much contemplation and logistical planning about how to gather Randy Michael's belongings and transport his remains back to Minnesota, Randy and I decided to drive to Colorado. We departed on Thursday, July 20. My sister Kathie; Randy's aunt Jane and her partner, Jeff; and our daughters flew out to meet us on Friday.

Despite our exhaustion and grief, the fourteen-hour car ride provided us with a sacred space for privacy—to converse, shed tears, reminisce, plan, and pray together for the challenging times ahead. As we exited the highway near Randy Michael's Denver apartment, I saw a homeless man sitting by the roadside. Unexpectedly, I thought, *Well, I suppose I will never have to worry about him being homeless.*

Then I glanced up toward the sky, and a breathtaking rainbow caught my eye. To me, it was a sign of hope and God's love, mercy, grace, faithfulness, protection, and renewal. Our sudden loss created profound grief that we would never see our son alive again in the present world, but that rainbow—and many other signs—brought a sense of peace. This was the first of many signs that made it so I would never again need to wonder where Randy Michael was or if he was all right.

We had planned to view Randy Michael's body on Friday at the mortuary, but delays in obtaining his body from the coroner's office meant the viewing needed to be postponed until Saturday afternoon.

We picked up our family from the airport, then made our way to Randy Michael's apartment to sift through his belongings and pack them up. It was surreal to collect his possessions without him there. When he had entered treatment in Florida in March, I had naively believed he would complete his program in three months, transition to a sober house, return home, resume college, and flourish in life.

Walking into his apartment building, my heart clenched within my chest, yearning for his presence at every turn. I couldn't shake the feeling that he would be meeting us in the lobby with his handsome smile, enveloping me in a warm hug, and saying, "Hey, Mom. Look at this amazing coffee bar! I love living here. There's a burrito shop I like. . . ."

Instead, the property manager who was expecting us, shyly, kindly, and quietly led us to his apartment and opened the door. En route, she tried to prepare us for what we would see, but how do you truly prepare to see the place where your son ended his life?

We were met with clothes scattered all over the floor, disorderly belongings, vacant floorboards, and an empty bedroom. The cleaning crew had removed soiled and damaged items like the bed, the frame, and some of the floorboards. Adjacent to the kitchen behind a wall that didn't go quite to the ceiling stood his makeshift recording studio. A note on the bathroom mirror read,

"If God brings you to it, God will bring you through it." I have had the same quote posted in my office since 2012.

There was also a handwritten Post-it Note on the mirror: "57 days hard, then home 7/07/21." It signified his plan to return home by August 29, 2021, aiming to promote his music at the state fair. All I could do was cry and make empty wishes. I wished he had believed that God would bring him through that July 16 evening. I wished he would have kept going hard for fifty-seven days, then come home. I wished I had been there with him on that dark evening to assure him everything would be okay. My wish list was never-ending.

Our family helped Randy and me sift through our son's belongings, and by Saturday morning, we wrapped up our tasks at the apartment and turned in his keys. Then we headed to the mortuary for our scheduled viewing with the priest. The funeral home had suggested bringing a hat for Randy Michael's head, so we chose his beloved SWAT hat.

Father Chris Marbury awaited us at the mortuary. He was a young, tall, and slender priest with beautiful, calming blue eyes. His demeanor was gentle and peaceful, and his presence immediately reassured us. Upon entering the area adjacent to the viewing room, we met the comforting young woman who had prepared Randy Michael for our viewing. Her name was Corey. Randy's youngest brother who died in the plane crash was named Corey. Then Corey told us that her dad's name was Randy. Strange that someone who would be involved in a very intimate and immediate part of our life would share the same names as those we had dearly loved and lost.

My inexplicable need to see Randy Michael's hands had continued through the week. We gave Corey the hat requested by the funeral home, and she told us she would be back in a minute. When she returned, she gently and sorrowfully explained that because Randy Michael had not been discovered for nearly forty-eight hours, his hands had started to decompose, so the mortuary had been forced to cover them with gloves.

Cautiously and with great hesitation, we slowly made our way into the small room where Randy Michael's body lay. Corey explained what we were about to see, but nothing could have prepared us for what we were going to feel.

The rush of emotions remains indescribable. My mind was flooded with countless thoughts. Our son didn't look like our son. There he was, lying on a gurney, wearing his SWAT hat that we just delivered, dressed in a random T-shirt, hands gloved and crossed on his lower belly, the remainder of his body covered by a green and blue plaid sheet. Logically, I knew it was his body, but he did not look or feel like the beautiful son I knew.

Weeping, I kissed his cheek and held him close. He was stiff and cold, so different from his warm, lively self. He always had the softest skin. I used to jokingly call him "hot hands" for his perpetually warm touch. He looked swollen and remarkably different. I could see a version of him, but not the real him. Despite the stark contrast, I am grateful for the viewing and the advice to bless him. Even as I write about it now, it feels surreal. I understand it but accepting this as our reality remains a constant struggle.

Eventually, we collected ourselves and formed in a U-shaped arrangement around Randy Michael's right side. I stood near his head with my hand on his arm, then Randy and our daughters, then my sister, then Jane and Jeff. The priest was at the end standing next to Randy Michael's feet.

I looked at Father Marbury and asked, "What should we do?"

His eyes filled with compassionate tears, and he said, "I've never done this, so you just let me know when you're ready, and we'll begin."

After a moment, I said, "Okay, let's begin."

Father Marbury conducted readings, blessed Randy Michael's body, and we all prayed together. As he concluded, Father Marbury said, "Jesus, take care of Randy Michael; Jesus, take care of Randy and Heather; Jesus, take care of Brooke, Sabrina, and Anna. Jesus, take care of our extended family. . . . Jesus, take care of it all."

It was a poignant prayer—one I knew I would hold onto in the days and years to come.

"Jesus, take care of it all."

Before departing, we bid one final goodbye to Randy Michael. Knowing my strong desire to see his hands, my family asked if I wanted a picture with my hands holding his. I was sad that he had to have gloves on, and I worried it might seem odd to take a photo. However, I realized it was a now-or-never moment and there isn't a "right" way to do these types of things, so Jane took a picture.

An Unexpected Detour

Sorting out Randy Michael's affairs included dealing with his two cars, the Nissan Leaf and his prized 2005 Corvette. The T-top Corvette had been a source of immense joy for Randy Michael during his final months and was also his way of connecting with his dad and grandfathers. My dad is a devoted car enthusiast, and Randy's father—whom Randy Michael never had the chance to meet—had a deep affection for Corvettes.

On Sunday, we headed toward the mountains in a caravan of cars to return the leased Nissan to the Boulder dealership.

Randy and Sabrina drove the Corvette for fun, while Anna and I drove the Nissan. Kathie had our car, and Jane and Jeff rode in their rental car.

Randy led the way, visibly enjoying the drive, while I struggled to keep pace in the electric car. At one point, Jane, Kathie, and I followed directions from our mapping system to exit the highway, but Randy kept going! When he arrived at the Nissan dealership ten minutes after everyone else, he said that his GPS app had instructed him to keep going. That longer route had taken him on a journey past Randy Michael's former workplace, the place where Randy had visited him during the COVID-19 shutdown, and the University of Boulder campus. It even took him past the parking lot where Randy had taught Randy Michael to ride his motorcycle before leading him back to the dealership.

It was an unusual but deeply touching experience for Randy. We believe Randy Michael's presence guided this final ride with his dad, visiting places they held dear in the car that he loved.

Searching for Jesus

In the weeks and months to come, Randy was able to access Randy Michael's computer and phone, and it provided us an enlightening view of our son's final days.

We believe Randy Michael's last use of marijuana was on July 6 or 7. Physical withdrawal peaks within a week to ten days after stopping, but psychological effects often intensify during that same period. Depression and insomnia are common as the body adjusts to functioning without THC. We will never have the exact answer, but what we do know is that THC had changed his brain, disrupted his homeostasis, caused psychosis, and altered his thinking, sleep, perception, and mood. We firmly believe had he not used marijuana starting at the age of fifteen, Randy Michael would still be here today.

Less than half an hour before Randy Michael's last text message, he had searched for images of Jesus three different times. He took the images he found and put one as his screensaver on his computer and another on his phone.

His last journal entry to himself was, "Can I live for Jesus . . . Can I?"

When authorities found Randy Michael in his apartment, his Bible was open to the book of Amos, an Old Testament book that addresses social, moral, and religious issues prevalent in ancient Israel while emphasizing the need for justice, righteousness, and true devotion to God. Next to him lay his rosary and a handwritten note that said, "I'm Sorry," placed on his right side.

We believe Randy Michael was seeking Jesus. Remember Father Marbury's prayer while blessing Randy Michael's body? "Jesus . . . take care of it all."

We are deeply convinced that Jesus did just that. We firmly believe Randy Michael wanted to be with Jesus. In his pain and suffering, we trust that God called him home. Despite the heartbreaking circumstances, we often find slivers of silver linings that bring us ongoing peace.

CHAPTER 14

GOODBYE, MY LOVE

The Funeral and the Eulogy I Wish I Had Written

A few weeks later, we gathered to remember Randy Michael at Saint Mary of the Lake Catholic Church in White Bear Lake, Minnesota. Despite the lingering shadow of COVID-19, friends and extended family showed up to the church for the visitation and his funeral Mass at the very place where we had baptized our son twenty-one years earlier.

We held the visitation on August 9, 2021, in the church's gathering space, which doubled as a calm and quiet place to bring our young and rambunctious children if they were disrupting Mass. It was also the backdrop for many happy events that were woven into our family's story. Having the visitation in this space brought us comfort.

I was overwhelmed in ways I had not anticipated when I stepped into the gathering space. Randy Michael's urn rested near the baptismal font surrounded by an ocean of exquisite flowers from our extended family and friends. The beauty stirred so many emotions and starkly reminded me of the harsh reality—I was attending my own son's visitation and funeral. I wish someone had prepared me for this moment, but perhaps there's no way to brace oneself for that kind of surreal, yet palpable pain.

Our church was filled with compassionate friends, family, and young souls who knew Randy Michael, and the hours slipped by in a blur of greetings and shared condolences.

I couldn't help but wonder: Does Randy Michael see this? Does he know how many people loved him? I often say, if love could have saved him, he would be here with us now! But I trust he was present, just in a different way than we can fully comprehend.

The line of mourners steadily wrapped outside the entry to the church, snaked down the center aisle, and then turned up the side aisle where they could greet our family and offer condolences and support. The love and solidarity extended to us are forever etched into our hearts. We are endlessly indebted to family and friends for their unwavering assistance, not just in those initial days, but also in the ensuing months and years that have followed. Their support remains a guiding light through our grief to this day.

Though I had asked Brooke to write Randy Michael's eulogy a week before his funeral, I was overcome by a need to write it myself. Perhaps it was a response to the loss, a way to grasp at some semblance of control amid the uncontrollable.

I aimed to honor Randy Michael thoughtfully while honestly addressing the circumstances surrounding his passing; we wanted people to know that Randy Michael had been suffering. I initially asked a friend to read the eulogy on my behalf, but he felt it was too personal and urged me to read it myself. Before walking up to the podium, I prayed for the Holy Spirit's strength and the Virgin Mary's support to get me through this.

In my left hand, I held Randy Michael's rosary, which had

been by his side at his death. Our daughter Sabrina walked next to me and stood by me in case I faltered. Miraculously, I made it through the entire eulogy without breaking down. It was an extraordinary moment, and I felt supported by something greater than myself every step of the way. And I felt sure that Randy Michael approved what I had to say.

Randy Michael's Eulogy

"Yes, the truth is, I don't wanna die an ordinary man."

Randy often sent us songs he liked or related to, and this is a line from a song he sent this past spring.

Randy did not die an ordinary man; his whole life, he was extraordinary, but he didn't know it—extraordinary means to go beyond what is usual, regular, or customary. Randy was extraordinary from the day he was born until the day he died. Physically, he was a Paul Bunyan–sized baby, and near his end, he towered over six feet, three inches. Mentally, he lived largely and had gigantic-sized dreams, goals, and aspirations.

In twenty-one years, Randy lived a lot of life to the fullest. He could be the sweetest, wisest, most thoughtful, kindhearted, hardworking, funny, and entrepreneurial-type spirit. At the same time, he could also be independent to a fault, defiant, anxious, lonely, impulsive, impatient, and prone to fixation. Throughout his childhood and young adulthood, these qualities brought both extreme joy and difficulty into our home, but they also allowed him the ability to venture west, get his residency, live independently, and start a clothing company and even a web consulting company. Pretty impressive for being just twenty-one years old!

Randy always knew what he wanted and loved to share his dreams, thoughts, and creative ideas. Randy had a great desire to be "normal" and accepted, but often did not do things conventionally. It wasn't that he wanted to be difficult; rather, he looked at things from his perspective. As a free spirit, he accepted others and spread joy and laughter to many, some of whom we will never know. One example was that he started volunteering at The Good Shepherd Parish in Denver, and we were told he had a welcoming smile as he held the door and greeted those returning to Mass after the pandemic.

After learning of Randy's tragedy, we traveled to Denver where he had recently moved. We were able to see his studio apartment, all that he was working on, and his dreams and goals on paper. Ideally, he wanted to be a music artist with a clothing line making lots of money. He wanted to get married, have a beautiful wife, and a family, heal his inner pain, and be successful. He was working like a fiend to achieve this and make ends meet but was also suffering from a long-standing struggle with mental health and, consequently, substance abuse. In March, he had entered a dual-diagnosis treatment center in Boca Raton, but after just a few hours, he had a change of heart and in an extraordinary fashion, left the treatment center and made his way back to Denver. On his own, he found a new therapist and psychiatrist for regular visits. We knew he needed more intense treatment, but he wanted to do it his way. After several weeks, we saw progress and in the last couple of weeks of his life, his demeanor had shifted. He was less argumentative, he was taking more responsibility for his actions, and he was appreciative, reflective, and loving.

We supported and encouraged Randy Michael from afar and with guarded hearts. We offered to visit him over the Fourth of July, but he wanted us to wait until August. He just accepted a new job in auto loan financing beginning in August, and we thought things were looking up.

Randy was returning to his faith, and we believe he was working on his substance use. However, as clarity and reality settled in, we think his depression and anxiety increased, and he became overwhelmed as he reflected on his actions and their consequences over the past few months.

His last text stated: "My attitude with the music and everything has been way too self-righteous. I am done with the music. I'm quitting weed for good and want to surround myself with healthy and happy people. This has been too much for me and you guys. I have been running from my past mistakes and I think it's time that I own up and start living a good life. Love you." Remember, he was impulsive, impatient, and hurting, and just forty-three minutes later he texted, "I love you and am sorry for everything. I love dad and the same for him. I wish I would have been a better person."

Then, in an instant, he was gone.

Randy did not die an ordinary man. He was extraordinary in every way. Nothing about him was usual, regular, or customary. In his short life, he made many extreme decisions, both good and bad. He walked in darkness and light. In the end, he owned his actions, said he was sorry, and shared his love not only with us but with many others. He returned to us for just a moment, and then it seems Jesus called him home to end his pain and suffering. That is extraordinary.

Randy, we wish you were here, and we miss you. We

will miss sitting next to you and discussing anything and everything—your silliness, wisdom, creativity, handsome smile, and compassionate heart. We will miss all the things that should have been. We don't understand, and we will always question. We will look forward to seeing you again when the time comes. We know you were welcomed by the loving arms of Jesus and so many others who have gone before us. We will continue to be the best parents we can be to your sisters. We will continue to seek peace, try to find joy, and, with the help of God's grace, work to be nothing short of extraordinary ourselves. We love you.

What We Know Now

What I expressed in Randy Michael's eulogy remains true. He struggled with mental illness, often resorting to self-medication, primarily using marijuana, and occasionally experimenting with substances like mushrooms.

However, while we initially believed Randy Michael was seeking relief through self-medication to manage a mental illness, hindsight has given us a different perspective. Given the knowledge and similar storylines we have uncovered, we are much more certain now that his adolescent substance abuse damaged his brain and led to his mental illness and his suicide.

Before Randy Michael's passing, we had obtained access to one of his many email accounts and witnessed a relentless job application spree—an average of three applications per day for weeks. His habit of changing passwords frequently, late-night texts containing cryptic notions about becoming "Big" enough to need secure communication, and his disturbed sleep patterns triggered a growing concern, while his grandiose ideas and erratic behavior indicated a declining mental state.

After his passing, we were able to explore the content of Randy Michael's phone and computer, and from his journals, photos, and videos, it became apparent that his daily drug of choice was marijuana.

We delved into every available piece of information, scouring items collected from Randy Michael's apartment, hospital records, autopsy details, and toxicology reports. Eventually, we gathered a comprehensive insight into his thoughts, activities, behaviors, physical well-being, and routines over his final couple of years, and especially the last eight months of his life.

Around three months after Randy Michael passed, a dear friend shared an article from *People* magazine that detailed the life of Johnny Stack—a life cut short by suicide linked to the use of high-potency THC products beginning at age fourteen. That article helped us begin to grasp what had happened to our son. Thanks to the efforts of Johnny's Ambassadors, the nonprofit established by John and Laura Stack, we have gained invaluable insights into the changes we witnessed in our son over the years.

Throughout this book, I have shared some of the insights we have gained about the dangers of marijuana use, especially on young brains. I have shared information from multiple research studies that show marijuana is addictive[72] and can lead to mental issues, including psychosis.[73] Knowing what I know now, I would write and deliver a very different eulogy for my son.

---

72 D. Ramesh et al., "Marijuana Dependence: Not Just Smoke and Mirrors," *ILAR Journal* 52, no. 3 (2011): 295–308, https://doi.org/10.1093/ilar.52.3.295.

73 Y. Hasegawa et al., "Microglial Cannabinoid Receptor Type 1 Mediates Social Memory Deficits in Mice Produced by Adolescent THC Exposure and 16p11.2 Duplication," *Nature Communications* 14 (2023), https://doi.org/10.1038/s41467-023-42276-5.

The Eulogy I Wish I Had Written

If I were to rewrite my eulogy for Randy Michael today, most of it would remain the same, but I would add words to warn every listener of the dangers I did not recognize until it was too late. Here is what I want everyone who came to mourn my son to know:

Regrettably, Randy's first encounter with marijuana began at the tender age of fifteen. By the time he turned sixteen, he was diagnosed with a cannabis use disorder. Marijuana is addictive. His early and frequent usage swiftly led to severe consequences on his mental well-being. Anxiety, depression, and suicidal thoughts started after he started using. Not only was Randy smoking, but he was also dabbing and vaping. By the fall of 2019, he suffered what we believe was his initial psychotic episode. He became convinced that his workplace was connected to the mob, and documented evidence reveals he heard distressing voices as well.

Despite intermittent attempts at "tolerance breaks," in March 2021, Randy Michael experienced full-blown psychosis. While shifting in and out of this state, he requested to go to treatment "…while he still had his brain." He agreed to go to treatment at a dual-diagnosis treatment center. Unfortunately, his stay lasted an hour or so due to severe withdrawal. Against our wishes, he returned to Denver convinced he could get sober on his own. He found a therapist and psychiatrist and had regularly scheduled appointments. We knew this wasn't enough and desperately wished we could have provided him with the care and support he needed within a secure and locked dual-diagnosis facility where he could not leave.

Experiencing suicidal thoughts in April, Randy Michael reached out for help. The police arrived and put his registered gun that was in his pants pocket away in his personal safe. They escorted him to the hospital. However, due to a lack of beds, he was discharged without receiving a diagnosis or any suggested follow-up care within twenty-four hours.

Over the following weeks, we noticed glimmers of hope. In the final stretch of his life, a noticeable shift occurred in his demeanor. He was less argumentative, he took responsibility for his actions, and he was deeply appreciative of his upbringing and for the love for our family. We supported Randy Michael with guarded hearts. We offered to visit him during the Fourth of July, but he said he planned on coming home in August. He seemed optimistic and even had a new job lined up in auto loan financing. We were hopeful for his future.

We didn't know, but hyper spirituality can be a sign of psychosis. In 2020, Randy Michael confided in me, sharing his experiences of conversing with both God and the devil. Thankfully, toward the end of his life, he rekindled his Catholic faith, regularly participated in Mass, and even attended Confession on July 13.

Three weeks before his passing, Randy Michael had been prescribed Adderall. This may have amplified his episodes of mania, depression, and anxiety. Maybe he was overwhelmed as he confronted the consequences of his past actions while working on his sobriety. It is also possible that an acute brain episode triggered auditory hallucinations, suggesting he end his life. His prolonged use of marijuana severely impacted the frontal lobe of his brain, leading to compromised impulse control and a lack of judgment, especially amid a somber, dark, sleepless moment. We will never know exactly what happened, but we know his brain was not working right, its growth and development hijacked by his marijuana use.

Weeks after he passed, we received his autopsy and toxicology reports. Wanting to know everything I possibly could about my deceased son, I read each report from beginning to end. One thing that surprised me on his autopsy was a finding that he had a mild thickening of his aorta at the age of twenty-one. That was likely due to his heavy use.

His toxicology report revealed that he had low levels of THC and alcohol in his system when he passed. Low levels indicate he was trying to quit because THC stays in the system for many days and had he used it recently, his numbers would have been higher. As clarity and reality began to set in, we believe several factors might have contributed to his suicide. We've learned that marijuana withdrawal is an undeniable reality. Between days three to five of abstinence, and again around days ten through fourteen, individuals often grapple with significant physical and mental challenges. Withdrawal induces heightened anxiety, depression, and a profound sense of despair, frequently resulting in insomnia. Intriguingly, most suicides occur after midnight. Randy Michael was experiencing insomnia alongside a body and mind not functioning right from his marijuana use, compounded by depression, anxiety, and psychosis; the odds were overwhelmingly against him. Oh, how we wish he could have held on for just a few more hours.

In a heartbreaking moment, he was gone. Sadly, marijuana gradually ravaged Randy Michael's brain and claimed our son over time.

The rest of his eulogy would remain unchanged. And it would still end with these words:

"We will continue to seek peace, try to find joy, and, with the help of God's grace, work to be nothing short of extraordinary ourselves. We love you."

> ### *You Need to Know*
>
> Marijuana use can cause an increased risk of myocardial infarction and stroke. The heavier the use, the greater the likelihood of an adverse event.[74] At the age of twenty-one, Randy Michael should never have had a thickening of his aorta. Not only that, when he went to the emergency department in March 2021, Denver Health told him that his lungs were damaged, which likely was due to his excessive marijuana use[75] and that he needed to decrease his smoking.

---

[74] Abra M. Jeffers et al. "Association of Cannabis Use with Cardiovascular Outcomes among US Adults," *Journal of the American Heart Association* 13, no. 5 (February 28, 2024), https://doi:10.1161/JAHA.123.030178.

[75] ScienceDaily, "How Long-Term Cannabis Use Can Damage Lungs," February 3, 2022, https://www.sciencedaily.com/releases/2022/02/220203192317.htm.

CHAPTER 15

LOVE OF SCIENCE

THC and Brain Development

Randy and I had never been political advocates, but in 2023, as our home state of Minnesota was pursuing legal recreational marijuana, we began actively working against the move with Smart Approaches to Marijuana, Minnesota. We even journeyed to the state capitol to voice our reservations. Although our state did legalize cannabis for recreational use for people twenty-one and older, and the widespread belief is that cannabis is safe, we will continue to tell our story and share a myriad of studies showing the opposite to be true.

A glance at the dictionary reveals that safety, fundamentally, means that a product or action is free from harm or risk. In its essence, today's marijuana does not align with this definition given that it primarily contains the psychoactive and intoxicating component, THC at a greater potency than ever.

Throughout this book, I have provided information about marijuana and the latest research into its effects on physical and mental health. In this chapter, I dive a little deeper into some of those topics and offer even more scholarly studies so that you can research on your own.

Arm yourself with knowledge as our lawmakers bow to pressure from an industry that I'm convinced is putting profits over lives. As parents, we must battle even harder for the sake of our children, and we must begin by understanding what we are facing.

Cannabis and Hemp

Cannabis and hemp are the same species of plants. Both types contain cannabinoids, which are chemical components that act as messengers in the human body, interacting with the brain's natural endocannabinoid system. The two cannabinoids that get the most attention are CBD (cannabidiol) and THC (tetrahydrocannabinol). Technically, both CBD and THC are psychoactive, but CBD is not intoxicating while THC is the intoxicating component responsible for the feeling of being high.

Legally, hemp must contain less than 0.3 percent THC and primarily consist of CBD. There are two types of cannabis plants—sativa and indica. Both are abundant with THC and have very little CBD (typically less than 0.10 percent).

Hemp can be used for industrial purposes, and CBD can be extracted from hemp and turned into foods, lotions, oils, capsules, and cosmetics. Proponents of CBD say it may aid with pain and sleep, reduce symptoms related to some mental health disorders, relieve certain cancer-related symptoms, have neuroprotective properties, and benefit heart health. The key word is "may." Currently, there is not enough evidence to prove that CBD is beneficial in all those areas. The Food and Drug Administration (FDA) has approved only one drug derived from CBD, Epidiolex, which is used to treat two rare childhood seizure disorders. It must be prescribed by a doctor, and the prescription is filled at a pharmacy, not a dispensary.

After copious amounts of CBD are extracted from hemp, chemists can alter its chemical bonds, creating hemp-derived THC-like analogs that are intoxicating. They are called derived psychoactive cannabis products (DPCPs). One example is Delta-8, which is about half as strong as THC Delta-9. Other examples are Delta-10, THC-P, THCV, and THC-O. There are over twenty-six different DPCPs.[76] These synthetic products can have the same detrimental effects on the developing brain as cannabis-derived THC Delta-9 can. DPCPs are sold primarily as vapes and edibles. Although they are not FDA-approved, they are now legally sold in many states due to loopholes in the Farm Bill passed in 2018.

The typical potency of marijuana in the 1960s and 1970s was 1 percent THC. By the 1980s, potency had increased to around 3 percent THC, and it rose to 5 to 10 percent THC in the 1990s. The THC content in cannabis products began an even greater upward trajectory starting in the mid-2000s. Presently, THC levels in marijuana products vary considerably, ranging from 15 percent to a staggering 99 percent, depending upon whether it's flower, concentrates, edibles, or dabs. Today's cannabis flower in its smokable form, consumed in a joint, bowl, bong, or blunt, ranges from 5 to 35 percent THC. Resins, concentrates, and dabs, which are extracted from the marijuana plant and vaped or heated to the point of combustion and inhaled, can vary from 30 percent to 99 percent THC. Edibles in the form of candies, cookies, gummies, powders, and tinctures vary in potency. Ten

---

[76] Matthew E. Rossheim et al., "Types and Brands of Derived Psychoactive Cannabis Products: An Online Retail Assessment, 2023," *Cannabis and Cannabinoid Research*, January 2024, https://doi.org/10.1089/can.2023.0266.

milligrams is a serving in Colorado, but one gummy might contain up to 50 mg.[77, 78]

Randy Michael began his journey with weed at fifteen in 2015, delving into high-potency Delta-9 THC derived from the cannabis plant. Like many parents, we weren't fully aware that today's marijuana is of much higher potency than the products being used when we were young.

THC and Endocannabinoids

In the 1990s, scientists made a pivotal discovery: our bodies naturally produce cannabinoids, known as endocannabinoids—"endo" signifying production within the body. These endocannabinoids bind with cannabinoid receptor cells scattered throughout the body. The two main ones are cannabinoid 1 (CB1) and cannabinoid 2 (CB2). CB1 receptors are abundant in the brain and central nervous system, and CB2 receptors are abundant in the peripheral nervous system. THC from the cannabis plant binds to these receptors and thus are activated when THC is consumed.

Anandamide is one of the major endocannabinoids that exists in the brain. Anandamide, which in Sanskrit translates to "pure bliss," is activated when we have positive experiences like exercising, eating a good piece of chocolate, enjoying a delicious meal, or having sex. Anandamide also serves to regulate movement, memory, appetite, and pain perception and contributes significantly to our body's equilibrium and homeostasis.

---

77 L. Cinnamon Bidwell, Renée Martin☐Willett, and Hollis C. Karoly, "Advancing the Science on Cannabis Concentrates and Behavioural Health," *Drug and Alcohol Review* 40, no. 6 (2021): 900–913, https://doi.org/10.1111/dar.13281.

78 M. A. ElSohly, S. A. Ross, Z. Mehmedic, R. Arafat, B. Yi, and B. F. Banaha, "Potency Trends of Delta9-THC and Other Cannabinoids in Confiscated Marijuana from 1980–1997," *Journal of Forensic Sciences* 45, no. 1 (2000): 24–30, https://pubmed.ncbi.nlm.nih.gov/10641915/.

As an endocannabinoid, anandamide readily binds to our CB1 receptors for the right amount of time and serves to activate other neurotransmitters, such as dopamine—the pleasure chemical in the brain. When a person consumes THC, it directly binds to and activates CB1 receptors, resulting in an excessive release of dopamine and creating a mimic effect of anandamide. Thus, the user experiences sensations of euphoria and a pronounced "high" feeling[79] (from the dopamine release) as well as disruptions in memory, movement, and appetite (from the mimic anandamide effects). However, these effects are not temporary. As THC persists or stays parked in CB1 receptors for an extended amount of time, it can create a prolonged period of disruption in functioning, as the brain's chemical balance is unsettled. Moreover, after repeated exposure to THC, the brain goes through a hijacking process that fosters a cycle of addiction and interferes with typical brain functioning (a neurobiological phenomenon that is common across all drugs of abuse),[80] and for youth, disrupts normal brain development. THC can also bind to CB2 receptors primarily located in the peripheral nervous system and immune cells and thus can interfere with normal functioning of these systems.

Brain Development

The brain develops from the back of the brain at the cerebellum to the front, the prefrontal cortex, and from the bottom to the top, reaching full maturity around age twenty-five for females

---

79 S. Chayasirisobhon, "Mechanisms of Action and Pharmacokinetics of Cannabis," *Permanente Journal* 25, no. 1 (March 1, 2021), https://doi.org/10.7812/TPP/19.200.

80 Alison C. Burggren et al., "Cannabis Effects on Brain Structure, Function, and Cognition: Considerations for Medical Uses of Cannabis and Its Derivatives," *American Journal of Drug and Alcohol Abuse* 45, no. 6 (2019): 563–79, https://doi.org/10.1080/00952990.2019.1634086.

and twenty-eight to thirty for males. Some studies reveal that teenagers who start using THC face irreversible damage to their developing brains. MRI imaging has shown that increased marijuana consumption in teens correlates with a thinning membrane in the prefrontal cortex, illustrating a documented physical alteration indicating actual brain damage.[81]

The prefrontal cortex, which develops last, is the part of the brain that helps with all the functions that assist in becoming productive and capable adults: impulse control, decision-making, time management, processing, working memory, self-awareness, emotional regulation, planning, perseverance and problem-solving. When cannabis comes in and disrupts that development, these skills do not flourish.

Adolescent Brain Development

Prior to adolescence, the brain goes through a phase of creating connections (synapses) between neurons, known as synaptogenesis. During adolescence, the brain undergoes a process to make communication between neurons more efficient. This process, called apoptosis, involves the pruning of synapses to refine neural connections. By stripping away unutilized pathways, the brain enhances specialization and the efficiency of communication. Additionally, the remaining pathways are insulated through a process called myelination, which creates faster and more efficient communication between synapses.

When THC enters the system of a developing brain, it disrupts this process: haphazard pruning can take place, an excessive number of healthy synapses may be eliminated by mistake, and

---

[81] M. D. Albaugh et al., "Association of Cannabis Use during Adolescence with Neurodevelopment," *JAMA Psychiatry* 78, no. 9 (2021): 1031–40, https://doi.org/10.1001/jamapsychiatry.2021.1258.

the insulation process may be harmed. These disruptions can contribute to a developing brain that does not work as efficiently as it should.[82] Marijuana users may wind up with decreased executive functioning skills and struggle with decision-making, time management, mood regulation, impulsivity, and interpersonal relations.[83]

Given the widespread presence of CB1 receptors throughout the brain's various regions, many areas of the brain are impacted when marijuana is used. Here are some examples: When THC binds to the amygdala, it can heighten feelings of paranoia and anxiety. This effect is significant because the amygdala plays a crucial role in emotion processing and threat detection. The interaction of THC with the prefrontal cortex influences cognitive functions such as decision-making, time management, and impulse control. This region is essential for executive functioning and when impaired can lead to increased impulsivity and poor judgment. In the hypothalamus, THC may cause hyperphagia, or the more commonly described munchies. In the hippocampus, THC can affect memory and learning, and in the neocortex, THC can affect how sensory information is interpreted, causing disordered thinking. Binding within the basal ganglia can impede reflexes and motor skills, potentially contributing to the heightened occurrence of traffic accidents. There are no tests or limits established to measure or judge driving impairment for individuals using THC, despite it being psychoactive and now legal in many states.

---

[82] A. Bara et al., "Cannabis and Synaptic Reprogramming of the Developing Brain," *Nature Reviews Neuroscience* 22 (July 2021): 423–38, https://doi.org/10.1038/s41583-021-00465-5.

[83] H. V. Curran et al., "Keep Off the Grass? Cannabis, Cognition and Addiction," *Nature Reviews Neuroscience* 17 (2016): 293–306, https://doi.org/10.1038/nrn.2016.28.

The bottom line is that the extensive distribution of CB1 receptors scattered throughout the brain underscores that THC's psychological and intoxicating effects significantly impact multiple brain functions and behaviors.

THC and Mental Health

The negative impact of THC on the brain is determined by several key factors. First, the age of initial use plays a crucial role—the younger an individual starts using, the more detrimental the effects tend to be.[84] Second, the frequency of use is a significant factor; frequent or daily usage heightens the risks.[85] Lastly, the potency of the substance matters. Higher potency levels increase the likelihood of brain damage.[86]

Randy Michael began using THC at the age of fifteen, maintaining regular, sometimes daily consumption. His preference for bud and flower (the smokable form), concentrates (vapes or dabs), and edibles created a perfect storm, significantly heightening the risks associated with his usage pattern. He began displaying signs of psychosis in the fall of 2019, marking just four years into his cannabis use. Previously, he hadn't exhibited psychotic behavior, but he did struggle with dysregulation, anxiety, and depression.

A longitudinal study conducted in Denmark demonstrates a direct correlation between the rise in cannabis potency, increased cannabis use disorder, and the heightened risk of schizophrenia. In Denmark, the incidence of schizophrenia surged from around

---

84 J. R. Alameda-Bailén et al., "Age of Onset of Cannabis Use and Decision Making under Uncertainty," *Peer J: Life and Environment* (July 3, 2018), https://doi.org/10.7717/peerj.5201.

85 G. Battistella et al., "Long-Term Effects of Cannabis on Brain Structure," *Neuropsychopharmacology* 39 (2014): 2041–48, https://doi.org/10.1038/npp.2014.67.

86 Stuyt, "Problem with the Current High-Potency THC Marijuana."

2 percent in 1995 to 8 percent in 2010, coinciding with the escalation in marijuana potency during the same period.[87]

Moreover, subsequent research from Denmark indicates another concerning statistic. In a fifty-plus-year study involving millions of individuals, findings suggest that 30 percent of schizophrenia diagnoses among men ages twenty-one to thirty are linked to cannabis use disorder. With cannabis usage growing rapidly in the United States among nineteen- to thirty-year-olds, a connection to schizophrenia could lead to disturbing trends in our society.[88]

A study published in *Psychological Medicine* in 2024 states that adolescents who use cannabis are at an 11 times greater risk for psychosis than those who do not. This is significantly higher than what it used to be, and many believe it could be attributed to higher-potency products.[89]

THC and Suicidal Ideation

In addition to inducing psychosis, high-potency THC products have been associated with an elevated risk of suicidal ideation. In a study of more than 280,000 adults ages eighteen to thirty-five, cannabis use was associated with an increased risk of suicidal

---

87 C. Hjorthøj, C. M. Posselt, and M. Nordentoft, "Development over Time of the Population-Attributable Risk Fraction for Cannabis Use Disorder in Schizophrenia in Denmark," *JAMA Psychiatry* 78, no. 9 (2021): 1013–19, https://doi.org/10.1001/jamapsychiatry.2021.1471.

88 National Institute on Drug Abuse, "Marijuana and Hallucinogen Use among Young Adults Reached All Time-High in 2021," August 2022, https://nida.nih.gov/news-events/news-releases/2022/08/marijuana-and-hallucinogen-use-among-young-adults-reached-all-time-high-in-2021.

89 André J. McDonald, Paul Kurdyak, Jürgen Rehm, Michael Roerecke, and Susan J. Bondy, "Age-Dependent Association of Cannabis Use with Risk of Psychotic Disorder," *Psychological Medicine* (May 22, 2024): 1–11, https://doi.org/10.1017/S0033291724000990.

ideation, plan, and attempt. This association remained whether the individual was also depressed or not. In this study, the risk was higher for women than for men.[90]

Since Colorado legalized recreational marijuana usage in 2014, it is the primary substance found in toxicology reports in youth suicides up to the age of 24, further underscoring its impact on mental health and well-being. The percentage of suicide incidents in which toxicology results were positive for marijuana has increased from 14 percent in 2013 to 29 percent in 2020.[91]

---

90 National Institute on Drug Abuse, "Cannabis Use May Be Associated with Suicidality in Young Adults," June 22, 2021, https://nida.nih.gov/news-events/news-releases/2021/06/cannabis-use-may-be-associated-with-suicidality-in-young-adults.

91 Colorado Center for Health and Environmental Data, "Suicide in Colorado: Demographics for Circumstances and Toxicology, Excludes Race," 2022, https://cohealthviz.dphe.state.co.us/t/HealthInformaticsPublic/views/COVDRSSuicideDashboardAllYearsExcludesRace/Story1?%3Aembed=y&%3Aiid=1&%3AisGuestRedirectFromVizportal=y.

CHAPTER 16

LOVE OF OUR CHILDREN

How to Help

I often reflect on what I could have done differently. I don't live in regret, but I do have regrets. I understand that I can't rewrite the past and that there would be no guaranteed positive outcome even if I could. While I don't dwell on these thoughts, I have written this book to share some insights that might help others who find themselves in similar situations.

As the commercialization and normalization of recreational marijuana continues to spread, I fear that more and more people may face the same devastating experience as ours. Tragically, many like our son, are misled by the marijuana industry that stands to profit from addiction presenting the drug as harmless and medicinal. Now it seems likely that the U.S. Drug Enforcement Administration will take steps to reclassify marijuana from a Schedule I drug to a Schedule III[92] further downplaying its risks.

---

[92] US Drug Enforcement Administration, "Drug Scheduling," 2018, https://www.dea.gov/drug-information/drug-scheduling.

What Can Parents Do?

Here are a handful of practical steps that parents can take to help their children avoid the dangers of a drug that is anything but safe. Failure to take a stand today imperils the well-being of our youth. Unfortunately, we know.

Trust Your Instincts

If something feels amiss with your child, listen to your gut. When your loved one isn't around, consider checking their room. Look under the mattress, the bed, in bathroom cabinets and drawers, and for secret hiding spaces. Our son created a hiding spot for his weed in the middle of a Harry Potter book by cutting out the center of the pages. Look for small signs like disassembled pens or nails (used for creating homemade smoking devices), lots of plastic baggies, or unfamiliar charging devices. We frequently discovered plastic baggies in the washing machine but were unaware initially that they were connected to marijuana.

We also found various chargers unrelated to our kids' gadgets—we didn't know it, but those were for vaping devices. Vapes come in diverse shapes—even a water bottle that sounds like it has a liquid in it can be a vape pen at the base of the straw. It appears your kids are drinking liquids, but they are vaping. Some parents assume their kids are vaping nicotine, but it could be THC. You must examine the cartridges to tell the difference.

Talk. And Listen

Initiate conversations regarding drug use at an early age and revisit them frequently. These conversations can arise organically, such as when a child falls ill and requires medication.

Use these moments to explain how medicine is prescribed by a doctor and must be taken only by the individual for whom it's intended and that it is purchased at a pharmacy. As children mature and become receptive to more nuanced discussions, maintain an open dialogue. Discuss drug-related themes presented in movies, music, and television shows. Simply listening to their perspectives can yield valuable insights, as they often have much to contribute.

Looking back, I regret trying to reason with Randy Michael after he started using. I wish I would have started discussing the dangers of all substances and how they impact the brain at a very early age. According to the science behind marijuana's impact on brain development, it's crucial to initiate conversations about its effects early and educate kids on their level of understanding. Listen attentively to what they share; you might be surprised by their knowledge.

Consider Testing

I wish we would have implemented regular drug testing for Randy Michael starting around age twelve—not because we suspected he was using, but to offer him a legitimate excuse if peers began to pressure him to try substances. He could have said, "I can't, I have to take mandatory drug tests at home." It gives your child a natural opt-out. Also, it is a way to say to your child, when they are younger, "Drug use will not be tolerated."

Furthermore, had we been consistently testing him, once he started using, it would have been easier for him to accept that we would continue to test him regularly because we already would have had a process in place. This is something we would have done for our daughters, too, even though they weren't using, simply to maintain fairness and consistency.

Create a Mission Statement

Consider crafting a family mission statement or family code when your kids are young. Outline your family's values and principles, displaying them openly in the home, perhaps in the kitchen where the family sees it every day. If we were to create a family mission statement or code with our kids today, it might look something like this:

> *Our family values God and faith and will treat others with respect and dignity. We acknowledge that life's fairness isn't guaranteed. Just because something is easy doesn't mean it's good, and just because something is hard doesn't mean it is bad. We prioritize honesty, accountability, and seeking forgiveness when necessary. We believe in mercy, granting forgiveness, and loving one another. We will not use substances or medications unless prescribed by a doctor. We will exercise, eat healthily, and have healthy social media, cell phone, and electronic device habits. We recognize our value as God's creation and will give our minds and bodies the greatest care and respect.*

In moments of conflict, a family code can serve as a powerful guide. It provides a framework to address behavior or resolve disagreements, emphasizing honesty, respect, and forgiveness. I realize now, looking back, that this code could have significantly guided Randy Michael and helped us to be better parents. It might have spared us from futile, heated arguments that left us all feeling frustrated, angry, and upset.

Advocate for Comprehensive Education

As parents across our nation confront the increasing possibility of their children encountering marijuana, we believe that comprehensive addiction prevention education must become ever more pronounced. Parents should advocate for schools to incorporate drug prevention courses from elementary school to high school.

Parents and their kids need to know about the varying and increasing levels of THC, the different types of THC products, the risks of adolescent marijuana use, and the links between marijuana and mental health problems. Lobby your school district to include such lessons in their drug education curriculum.

Know Your Kids' Friends—and Their Parents

Parents should ensure that the values they are teaching their children regarding substance use are the same values their kids' friends are learning from their parents. If your values do not align with the values of other parents in your kids' social circle, you will have a hard time enforcing your rules.

During our children's school years, we observed parents hosting gatherings for adolescents where they allowed them to use substances such as alcohol and marijuana. These parents thought they could provide a "safe" environment simply by confiscating car keys and cell phones. However, allowing adolescents to engage in such behavior fails to acknowledge varying predispositions to addiction or potential interactions between medications and substances. Offering a comfortable space for kids to party reinforces the notion that the substances themselves are safe and that driving (or arriving home) while drunk or high is the only danger.

All parents should know about the inherent risks associated with youth substance use and how those substances can affect the developing brain.

Advocate for Sensible Laws

Parents must engage with lawmakers at state and national levels to advocate for sound drug policies and increased investment in prevention, recovery, and treatment initiatives. They should also petition city councils, expressing opposition to the establishment of vape and marijuana dispensaries within their communities, thereby asserting local control over such matters.

Our home state of Minnesota does not allow for a city or county to opt out of marijuana dispensaries, which means we have the potential to have pot shops in every city and town in our state. But local governments still have some authority over how many dispensaries will be allowed in a locale, where dispensaries can be placed, and when and how cannabis can be used within city limits. Parents should become involved in making these decisions.

Recognize Signs of Drug Use, Suicidal Tendencies

Knowing that marijuana can lead to anxiety, depression, suicidal thoughts, and psychosis would have shed light on so much of our son's behavior. We often attributed his rudeness, aggression, and irrationality solely to his personality. That was a mistake. If we had understood the impact of marijuana, we could have better separated his actions from his personality and recognized the drug's influence on his behavior.

If you notice subtle signs of paranoia in a loved one, such as overanalyzing texts or questioning responses, it might be a concern. Hyper spirituality, sudden claims of divine connections, or extreme changes in character could also be indicators that a person may be suffering from psychosis. Giving away personal belongings, hints about not seeing you again, eating or sleeping more or less than usual, experiencing extreme mood swings, withdrawing from friends and family, or giving reminders that life is short could be signs that a loved one is considering suicide. We were unaware of these signs, and looking back, I wish we had been more knowledgeable and informed.

Know Mental Health Treatment Options

If I had comprehended the depth of Randy Michael's mental illness, I would have pursued commitment options in states with stricter laws. When Randy Michael admitted himself to Denver Health in April 2021, expressing suicidal intent and meeting every alarming criterion, I was shocked that he was allowed to leave. It amazes and dismays me that we allow individuals in mental distress to make critical decisions about their well-being.

As mentioned, Florida's Baker Act and Marchman Act allow for court-ordered commitments, but I did not know about those options when we took Randy Michael to Florida for treatment. If I had known, I could have pursued options to keep him there against his will.

I wish I had insisted on antipsychotic medication when he went to detox in Florida. Perhaps it would have brought him clarity and helped him stay at the treatment center. We'll never know, but it's frustrating to see how the systems and professionals often fell short with his care.

For parents with children over eighteen, it is imperative that you obtain a signed release of information form if your child is getting mental health care. This form grants access to health information and facilitates communication with doctors. Randy Michael always allowed us to speak with his care team, but at that time we didn't always know what signs to look for or what questions to ask.

Seek Professional Help

It's crucial that you find professional guidance for both you and your loved one. Thoroughly evaluate potential professionals—interview them, make sure your values align, and confirm they specialize in your loved one's needs. If substance abuse is involved, a licensed drug and alcohol counselor is invaluable. Research treatment facilities that are adept at addressing dual diagnoses for mental health and substance use concerns. Support groups can also be incredibly beneficial; finding the right fit might take time, but it's so worthwhile. Mar-Anon, Al-Anon, and Narcotics Anonymous are among the well-known options.

Above All, Love

Love should be at the forefront of every action when you have a loved one struggling with addiction. Establish firm boundaries rooted in care and concern for their well-being. Rather than judge their actions, ask yourself the why behind the action. There's usually a reason.

Catering to every desire, especially for a person with a substance use disorder, can often be harmful to them. But you must find ways to show respect and dignity, a balance between displaying love and setting necessary limits. Thankfully, in the last two months of Randy Michael's life, he found some peace. He didn't challenge our boundaries; we were on good terms, and he seemed content. We cautiously embraced those moments, fully aware of the potential that his attitude could change and of the reality that when dealing with addiction, there will undoubtedly be ups and downs.

Lean on your Higher Power during challenging times. Life isn't easy and believing you're navigating it with the help of a

Higher Power can offer immense strength. Personally, my Higher Power is Jesus; through Him, I find hope, even in the darkest moments.

We are committed to preserving our son's memory by sharing his story. We extend an invitation for others to join us in this endeavor. If you feel called to action, we encourage you to reach out and become a leader for Be Extraordinary, Be You—an initiative we launched that is dedicated to preventing youth marijuana use.

Writing this book has been a way of demonstrating my ability to keep hoping. It is my fervent hope that by sharing our journey, we can prevent use and spare others from needless pain. When addiction, mental illness, or suicide happens, riptides from a vast ocean of whys drag survivors down, drowning out any voice of reason or aid. Instantly, the world becomes very dark and silent.

We were fortunate. Our son left us a treasure trove of gifts—voicemails, texts, videos, photos, and journals of his personal journey while suffering from addiction. His records, although painful, are like a life preserver to us. Waves of *Why?* and regrets lap at our legs, but his gifts enlighten us and release us from drowning in agony. We now walk in peace, knowing we did the best we could with what we knew at the time . . . and for the love of ***others,*** we share all that we have learned.

EPILOGUE

LOVE REMAINS

Seeing Silver Linings

On the day after we learned of Randy Michael's death, one of our calls was to our priest, Father Talbot. He prayed with us and for us and helped us with logistical details. And he also advised us to seek out silver linings and avoid getting lost in the haunting labyrinth of what-ifs.

Those were words of profound wisdom. We have journeyed a few years past the phone call that changed everything and have discovered so many silver linings along the way. The specter of "what if" still rises into view occasionally, but we are encountering it less and less as we learn the art of forgiveness and letting go.

We grant ourselves forgiveness and extend it to Randy Michael. By forgiveness, I mean relinquishing the desire for a different or better yesterday—a concept eloquently expressed by John W. James and Russell Friedman in the Grief Recovery Method.[93] We

---

[93] John W. James and Russell Friedman, *The Grief Recovery Handbook, 20th Anniversary Expanded Edition: The Action Program for Moving beyond Death, Divorce, and Other Losses including Health, Career, and Faith* (New York: William Morrow, 2017).

keep in mind that the prospect of a better yesterday or alternative outcomes is futile. Dwelling on what-ifs merely conjures up endless, impossible scenarios, squandering time, and emotional and mental energy, with no guaranteed positive outcome.

Moreover, phrases like "silver linings," "bittersweet," and "dark gardens" have taken on profound significance for me. I've come to understand their depths during this period of tremendous turmoil and heartache. Even in profound suffering, immense beauty exists if you are open to perceiving and embracing it.

In addition, I have come to see "coincidences" and sightings in nature as evidence of Randy Michael's presence and that God is carrying us through our grief. I will share some of those moments here.

Randy Michael's final text stirred a sense of unease in my heart, although I hesitated to acknowledge it. A subtle sadness persisted even as we attended a gathering with friends by the lake that Saturday evening. I was lost in thought until I glanced up to notice a solitary monarch butterfly flitting by. It marked my first sighting of a butterfly for the summer.

The next morning, we were participating in an online Mass because Randy's sudden allergy attack prevented in-person worship. My attention drifted as I thought about Randy Michael, and then I spotted another monarch butterfly from our window. I noted its presence because we rarely see monarchs in our backyard.

Later that afternoon, I was immersed in a book that reminded me of Randy Michael while enjoying a tranquil pontoon ride on White Bear Lake. I closed the book and looked up in time to see another monarch butterfly passing by. Once again, I took note of it because I thought it was odd to see a butterfly out that far in the lake. And it was the third monarch butterfly I had seen in less than twenty-four hours.

Later, after we received the devastating news and after we heard Father Talbot's wise words, I remembered those butterfly sightings. Immediately, butterflies became a signal to me of Randy Michael's presence.

Brooke, our oldest daughter, returned home on Sunday, July 18. Although we had been concerned about Randy Michael since receiving his text early on Saturday morning, we did not call the Denver police to request a wellness check until Monday afternoon.

Looking back, I'm convinced there was a divine purpose in the timing. Brooke had been the last family member to see Randy Michael alive, and the thought of her grappling with the news of his death on her own is too painful to bear. I'm filled with immense gratitude that Brooke was by our side when we received the devastating news. Our shared presence provided much-needed support and solidarity during an incredibly challenging time.

We received news of Randy Michael's passing on Monday night and departed for Denver on Thursday. Before our departure, we busied ourselves tidying the house and caring for the lawn and our gardens, finding a sense of normalcy in the routine. Randy had been contemplating removing a near-dead rosebush outside of Randy Michael's window all summer. It was dry and thorny, lacking any leaves or buds. But as Randy watered the yard in the days after our son's death, he discovered two fresh, exquisite roses had bloomed from what had been a lifeless plant just days earlier.

Overwhelmed with emotion, Randy came inside, tears streaming down his cheeks. Filled with a blend of bittersweetness and hope, Randy told me about the roses. He perceived them as a poignant sign of resilience and ongoing life, and so did I. Ironically, that rose bush flourished the remainder of that summer and continues to do so today.

As I described in a previous chapter, I had a strong desire to see Randy Michael's hands when we viewed his body at the mortuary. Unfortunately, that was not possible, but before we left the viewing that day, I reluctantly agreed to allow Randy's aunt Jane to take a picture of me holding my son's gloved hands. That picture later became a treasure to me, and I'm convinced it is a message from our son, something seemingly coordinated by divine intervention.

When we returned home and began examining the belongings we had removed from Randy Michael's apartment, we discovered a piece of his journal from January 2021. The three-page entry detailed his short-term, long-term, and lifetime goals alongside some of his artwork, including a drawing reproduced in Photo 1. Randy Michael intended to use this drawing for one of his album covers. Pay attention to the time on the sketched clock face, with the minute hand pointing to the word "Forever," and the hour hand pointing to the word "Now." Below the clock, Randy Michael has written, "Mom+Dad+FAM+ME."

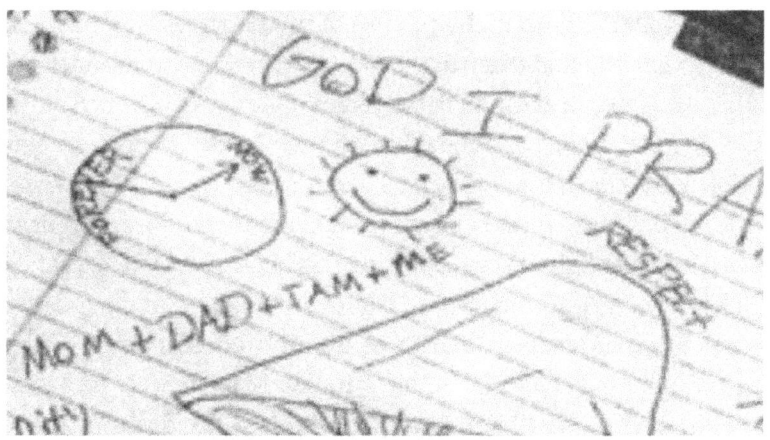

Photo 1. Randy Michael's intended album cover art

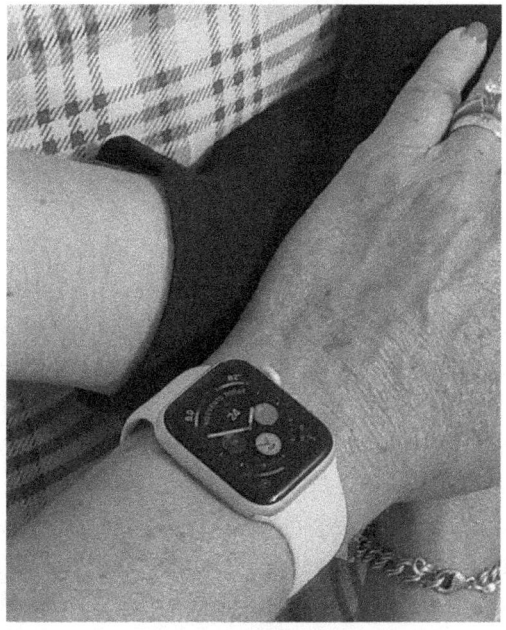

Photo 2. My hand on Randy Michael's

Now look at Photo 2, the picture of my hand resting on Randy Michael's gloved hand taken at the mortuary viewing on the afternoon of July 22. Note the position of the hands on my watch, which almost perfectly mirrors the hands on the clock that Randy Michael sketched.

Below the clock, Randy Michael had written "Mom + Dad + Fam + Me." That was the exact way we had arranged ourselves as we blessed his body right before capturing this photo at 1:50 p.m. that day.

The way our photo mirrored Randy Michael's sketch could not be just a coincidence. It had to be divinely coordinated. We had originally been scheduled to view his body on Friday at 3 p.m., but the viewing had been changed to Saturday at 1 p.m. I had been telling everyone of my deep desire to see my son's beautiful hands, and that is why Randy's aunt encouraged me to have this photo taken. I will forever be grateful that we took advantage of that now-or-never photo opportunity. Discovering that the photo of our hands mirrored Randy Michael's artwork gave us a profound message of hope, implying our eventual reunion and our son's enduring presence with us. God works in mysterious ways.

The day after viewing Randy Michael's body, we caravanned from Denver to Boulder to return his Nissan Leaf to the dealership. After completing that task, we headed up to Flagstaff Mountain, a spot Randy Michael had taken us more than once when we visited him in the summer of 2019. He held a special fondness for that lookout point.

I was exhausted by the past few days, and my heart ached for my son, feeling the injustice of his absence. Then a single monarch butterfly appeared. Its sudden presence stirred a sense of connection, once again making me feel our son's essence. It was the only monarch I encountered during our time in Colorado.

While we were in Denver, we also had to deal with Randy Michael's Corvette. Although we were attached to the car because we knew how much Randy Michael valued it, it needed extensive repairs and attention. So, we made the tough decision to return the car to the credit union that held his loan. We took several photos of the vehicle before we returned it and kept one of the personalized license plates that read, "LilRand."

After we returned to Minnesota, Jane noticed a striking detail in one of the photos, which had been taken on a beautiful sunny day with only a few faint clouds. Nothing was present overhead when we snapped the image shown in Photo 3. I believe the photo captured the image of something otherworldly; look closely at the black figure on the right side of the car hood and check out the close-up of that figure in Photo 4.

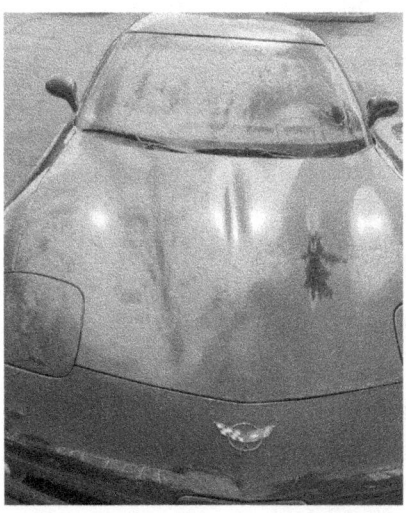

Photo 3. A mysterious black figure reflected in the hood of Randy Michael's Corvette

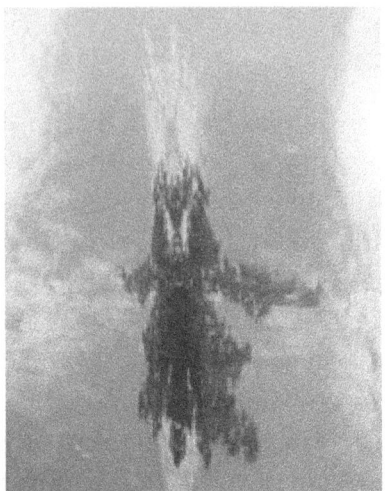

Photo 4. Silhouette suggests angelic and demonic forms

When we look at this image, we see a silhouette suggestive of a little person being lifted by what appears to be an angel from a darker demonic form. I often believe that a demon had a hold on Randy Michael in those very difficult months of his life. And I know that when he passed, he was saved by divine intervention. In the picture above, the angel figure bears an uncanny resemblance to a seraphim, which are beings often associated with purification and guiding souls toward the divine presence.

In another "coincidence," among the few pieces of artwork I preserved from our kids over the years, I have discovered some of Randy Michael's creations that bear a striking similarity to the darker imagery captured in the Corvette photo. Photos 5 and 6 are pictures of artwork Randy Michael made in 2008 and 2009, when he was nine and ten years old.

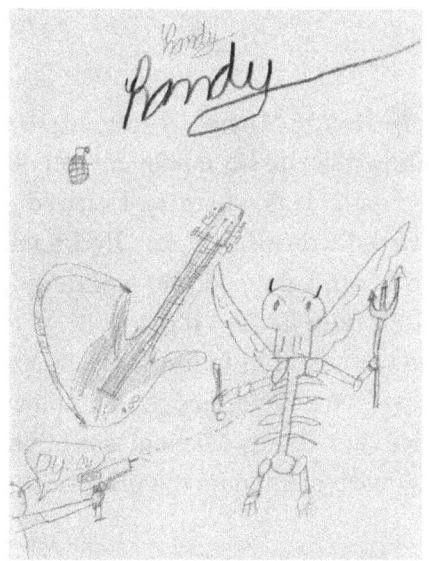

Photo 5. Shooting at a demonic figure

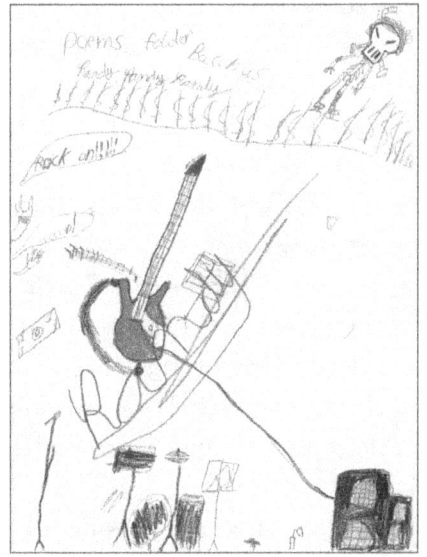

Photo 6. Demonic figure hovering over illustrations of music creation

A few days before Randy Michael's August 10 funeral, I felt a strong inner calling to write his eulogy myself. While Randy and the girls watched a movie downstairs, I retired to our room and began crafting what I wanted to share. By 1 a.m., I had finished.

As I wrapped it up, I paused and wondered, *Would Randy Michael approve? Would he find it fitting?*

Suddenly, the recessed lights in the perimeter of our ceiling blinked repeatedly—this never happens. I know it was a sign. It was a reassurance that Randy Michael was at peace with what I would say. I was overwhelmed by his presence.

I have always loved roses. We had only roses at our wedding, and they were even sprinkled atop our wedding cake. Before Randy Michael left our care, I would often say a Hail Mary prayer over him. In moments of distress and sleepless worry, I'd recite the Rosary, asking Mary to protect him, intercede, and bring our concerns to Jesus. In the Catholic faith, the rose is associated with Mary.

In preparation for the wake and funeral, my siblings and their spouses curated a bouquet of thirteen roses, representing the thirteen grandchildren on my side of the family. In the middle of twelve white roses stood one striking orange rose, symbolizing Randy Michael's vibrant spirit. He adored orange. The vase of flowers was placed alongside Randy Michael's urn and a photo of him at the altar.

The priest blessed the urn with holy water during the funeral, and I am positive that some holy water got on the roses. Following the funeral, our home was filled with beautiful flower arrangements, including the roses that were placed on my kitchen table where I could see them daily. Within six days, all the white roses wilted and drooped, but the orange rose remained fresh and upright, as you can see in Photo 7. Perfect! It even sprouted new leaves where thorns once were. It was a marvel to witness.

I was amazed by how this rose stayed beautiful and in perfect condition for well over a week. It sprouted new life, and for the second time since our son's passing, roses became a symbol for us. It seemed to affirm that Randy Michael had embarked on a new life with Jesus and reassured me that Mary had been watching over him all along, guiding him back to Jesus's loving embrace and making him whole and eternal.

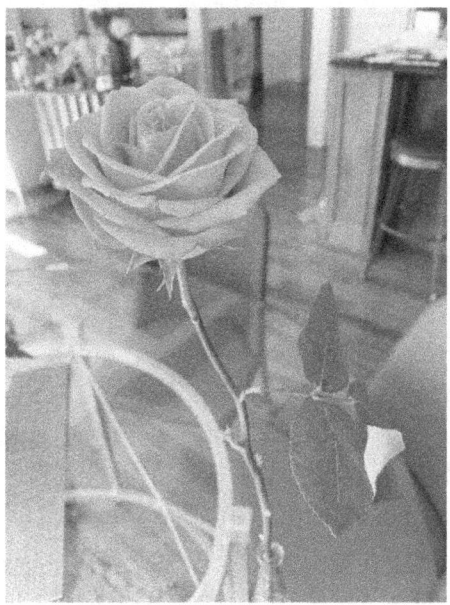

Photo 7. The orange rose remained vibrant for days

The rose from the funeral arrangement stayed beautiful for so long that I was even able to replant the stem and watch it continue to grow for weeks. Randy Michael's artwork also contained roses. Photo 8 is one of his pieces with a rose that we can relate to so much now. Beauty and pain. Bitter and sweet.

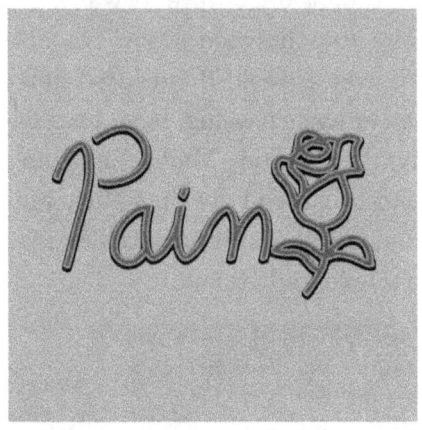

Photo 8. Randy Michael, age 20 used a rose in his artwork that seems to foreshadow the future

Butterflies have continued to appear in our lives unexpectedly, marking significant moments since Randy Michael passed away. While going through his computer files, we found a captivating butterfly design in his artwork. The design in Photo 9 was initially part of his clothing line release, and we were able to include the design in his funeral program and thank-you notes. Now it is the basis for the logo for our nonprofit organization, Be Extraordinary, Be You.

LOVE REMAINS

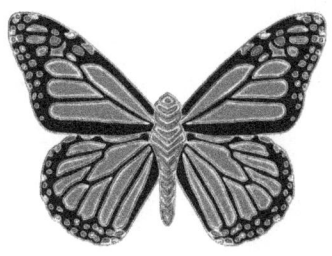

Photo 9. Randy Michael's butterfly design

In August 2021, Jane discovered a monarch caterpillar in her garden, which she generously brought to our house. Within days, we had the remarkable opportunity to witness its transformation. I happened to be walking by right as it spun into a chrysalis. The vibrant caterpillar, once hanging from the lid by a tiny little thread, started spinning and evolved into a breathtaking bright green cocoon adorned with intricate gold patterns in a matter of minutes. After about ten days, a magnificent monarch butterfly emerged—for us, a poignant symbol of our son's journey from this life to the next.

On September 8, 2021, before a walk with Alec's mom, I asked Randy Michael for a sign that he would be with us. We walked for two miles without mentioning Randy Michael. When we started discussing him, guess what flew by? Of course, a monarch! I believe it was a powerful and timely sign that my son was with us at that very moment.

In March 2022, during a trip to Fort Lauderdale, Florida, a monarch landed by me while we waited outside a smoothie shop. I have been visiting that area for more than thirty years and have never seen a monarch. As I attempted to photograph the butterfly, it circled me three times before taking flight.

On the first anniversary of Randy Michael's death, Randy's aunt Joye and uncle Jon and their grandchildren visited our house while the girls and I were driving two hours away to pick up our new grief puppy, Boots. The kids spotted a Hulk doll in our garage that had once belonged to Randy Michael. Randy offered them the doll and a couple of model cars that had belonged to to him as well.

After making the offer, Randy grew concerned that I might be upset about him giving Randy Michael's toys away. However, as he handed over the cars, a butterfly appeared, hovering overhead. It fluttered around Randy three times, a profound moment that seemed to signal Randy Michael's approval. Moved to tears, Randy was reassured that he had made the right decision.

These encounters may sound simple, but their frequency feels more than mere coincidence. Randy Michael's fondness for butterflies in his artwork, and the consistent appearance of monarchs after his passing, resonate deeply with us as a powerful sign of beauty, transition, and his ongoing presence.

In the summer of 2022, I stumbled upon three monarch caterpillars and seven black swallowtail caterpillars. It was the first time in our fifteen years in this house that I had ever seen caterpillars on our front porch. I placed them in a butterfly cage and watched them go through their incredible transformation. When they were ready, we released them.

This newfound tradition of nurturing caterpillars into butterflies holds a deeper meaning for our family, as it reflects the concept of the butterfly effect, where seemingly small events lead to significant consequences. This notion resonates with Randy

Michael's journey. Seemingly small decisions ultimately caused him great harm, altered his brain, and deeply affected our lives. His butterfly designs and the consistent presence of butterflies since his passing signify his transition to a better place, a symbol of transformation and restoration to health.

In the wake of Randy Michael's passing, Randy channeled his grief into creating a beautiful garden in our backyard, nurturing the soil, planting five rose bushes, and cultivating various flowers that attract pollinators. He also constructed a new paved patio, pouring his heart and soul into this labor of love. The following summer gifted us the delight of a blossoming garden—vivid with blooming shrubs and perennials that painted the landscape.

Toward the end of September 2022, I found myself seated on our deck in the sunshine. A sudden inner urge nudged me to glance over at the rose bushes. When I did, a breathtaking sight unfolded before me: two monarch butterflies gracefully fluttering around the rose bushes. In these moments, I have felt Randy Michael's presence as a comforting and reassuring reminder of his spirit surrounding us. And I am so grateful.

Approximately two months following his passing, the Denver police returned his phones to us. Despite numerous attempts, Randy couldn't crack the security code on one of the phones, which was protected by a pattern lock. Each failed attempt resulted in the phone locking itself. He eventually resorted to purchasing a program to bypass the phone's security, but when he activated the program, a dire warning flashed on the screen, indicating that continuing would erase all data on the phone.

In a moment of desperation, Randy vocalized his plea aloud, saying, "Please God and Randy, help me unlock this phone!"

Summoning the courage to try again, he again tried the very first pattern he had ever attempted. Miraculously, the phone unlocked, and we were blessed to discover a treasure trove of video content captured by Randy Michael during the final nine months of his life. From the video on this phone, we discovered that he had been engulfed in delusions but convinced of his future as a renowned rap artist. The videos were originally intended to document his pathway to stardom.

However, the extensive footage revealed the stark duality of his existence—his relentless pursuit of success colliding with his deteriorating mental state. He appeared delusional, maintained a constant use of marijuana, and candidly discussed his psychosis and mental health struggles.

The unlocked phone held valuable answers, offering profound insights into the life of our cherished son. The divine intervention that granted access to this content remains an immeasurable source of gratitude.

In April 2022, I found myself submerged in intense despair, revisiting the difficult moments from the previous year when Randy Michael had been struggling with so much. I was engulfed in feelings of grief, anxiety, isolation, hopelessness, deep sadness, and a profound sense of being lost.

Unexpectedly, a life-altering message reached me from an unlikely source—the young son of a family I had helped to find a new home in the autumn of 2020. We had formed a bond during our house-hunting adventures, and the mother contacted me again in April 2022 to discuss an investment property. During our meeting, she unexpectedly handed me a collection of drawings created by her youngest son, then around four years old.

She told me that the boy had crafted the heartfelt drawings earlier that week and had asked his mother, "Who was the lady that helped us find our house?"

When she told him my name, he said, "Yes. These pictures are for her."

When asked why, he earnestly replied, "I made these for that lady who sold us our house because I don't want her to be sad; I want her to be happy. She just needs to be happy."

His mother handed me the drawings and recounted her son's heartfelt wish for my happiness. The drawings included a pair of crosses, rainbows, an eye, and a painting made with a toothbrush. His mother, who had not disclosed Randy Michael's death to their children, told me her son was not typically inclined toward art and had never created anything like this.

As she shared the drawings with me, she said, "I hope our son's drawings brought peace to your heart. Every night, I pray that God reveals his gift to share with the world. I didn't expect this, but God works in mysterious ways."

In those innocent drawings, so reminiscent of what my son might have created at that age, I sensed a message conveyed by Randy Michael that I indeed needed to be happy and to let go of my dismay and despair. That day became a pivotal moment in my journey through grief, and that little boy's artwork provided a profound indication that our son was at peace, close by, and that he wished for my peace as well.

As 2023 came to a close we experienced another significant sign. Since losing Randy Michael, we have headed to Florida to celebrate the holidays and be with my parents, who are snowbirds. As I mentioned, I have been going to Fort Lauderdale for thirty years. In the early years, shells were abundant, and my mom, sister, and I would spend hours upon hours collecting shells of all shapes and sizes. We had gallons and gallons of shells. However, about fourteen years ago, Fort Lauderdale began efforts to slow the erosion of the beaches, and it has become rare to find a shell of any decent size on the beach.

On our last beach day of 2023, I was walking in the shallow water, which was calm and glistening. My heart was relaxed and happy and I thought, *God and Randy Michael, if you are with me, send me a sign*. But I quickly retreated from that thought, saying internally, *No, no, I know you are with me, I don't need a sign*.

But when I looked down at my feet, I saw something was shining, gliding, and moving as the water caressed the sandy shore. I reached down to snatch it up and was surprised to retrieve a three-and-a-half-inch, perfectly intact conch shell! I could not believe my eyes.

My heart exploded with profound joy and gratitude. Randy Michael and God were listening! I know they sent that shell, which you can see in Photo 10. It now sits next to my Sacred Heart of Jesus photo where I start each day in prayer. I am convinced our loved ones who have passed are with us and never far away.

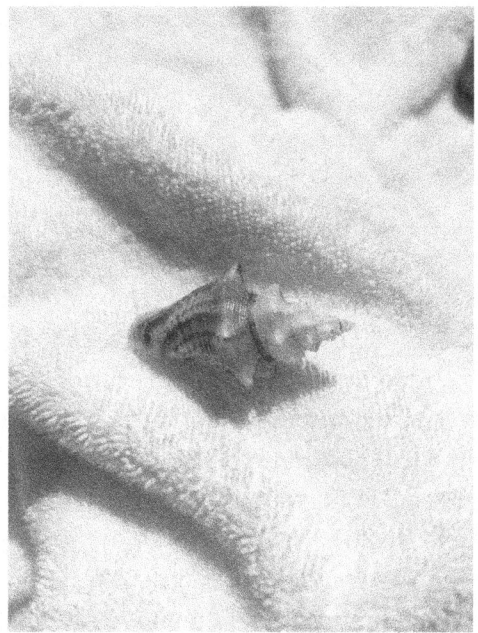

Photo 10. A beautiful shell reminds me of the presence of my son

We have a special friend who has the unique gift of being able to communicate with our son. I'll call her "Heidi." From the very first day we learned of our loss, Heidi has shared her wisdom and prayers and has been a pillar of support for our family. She has graced us by decorating our yard and delivering a cake on our son's birthdays, even though he asked her for fireworks. Heidi doesn't do fireworks, but it's funny that he would ask her to! Randy Michael loved fireworks!

You might wonder how this is possible, but as I said, she has the gift of communicating with those who have passed. Skeptics might not believe it, but there have been too many things she has shared with us that she couldn't have known. For instance, she conveyed a message to the girls from Randy Michael, using their nicknames, and said the message was from "Bubbee," Randy Michael's nickname when he was just a little one.

On January 5, 2024, Heidi texted me. It had been a while since we visited, and she shared that Randy Michael wanted me to listen to the song "Fall on Me" by Maverick City Music. I told Heidi I would add it to my playlist of hopeful songs for Randy Michael. We continued texting that day well into the evening.

That same evening, I learned devastating news about my dear friend's daughter Elena, who is the same age as our beloved Randy Michael. In 2019, Elena had a noncancerous tumor growing near her eye and brain, which required a craniotomy to remove. It was a painful, worrisome, and frightening experience. Elena did well and they were able to remove the tumor, but a craniotomy is a very serious procedure with a lengthy and emotional recovery.

Earlier that day, I had been judging a high school competition with Elena's mom, who told me Elena hadn't been feeling well. She was suffering from headaches, fatigue, sinus issues, nausea, and severe pain. That evening, sweet Elena went to the hospital, where our friend, a neurosurgeon, had ordered an MRI. The MRI showed that the tumor was back, and she had a severe sinus infection creating immense pressure on her brain. She was immediately admitted for IV antibiotics and a plan to remove the tumor.

Worried about Elena and still texting with Heidi, I stayed up later than usual, binge-watching the last season of *The Crown*. I went to bed around midnight. In one of my texts to Heidi, I asked her to convey a message to Randy Michael, telling him how much we love and miss him and requesting that he continue to watch over us. Exhausted, I climbed into bed and adjusted our dog, who was stretched out alongside me. I was feeling so sad and worried about Elena, questioning once again what life is all about. *Why does suffering exist?*

Once I settled in bed, I noticed my heart was beating irregularly. It wasn't a palpitation; it was a rapid flutter located in the center of my chest, not the intermittent rolling feeling that I have experienced previously from heart palpitations. This was different; it was consistent and lasted for at least a minute and a half. I wondered if I should tell Sabrina, who was in nursing school, so that if something bad happened, they would know to check my heart. That's how unusual and remarkable the feeling was. As quickly as it came on, it suddenly stopped. I breathed a sigh of relief and fell into a deep sleep, snoring myself awake the following morning.

My morning habit is to wake up, grab my phone, and head to the living room to start my day in prayer in front of a Sacred Heart of Jesus photo. Once I finish my prayers, I open my email to see what has come in overnight. This particular morning, there was a note from Heidi. The subject was: "I couldn't wait!"

January 6, 2024, 12:32 AM

Heather,

I got very excited about the idea of passing along a message so forgive me for sending this so late, but I wanted to report back lest my memory start to lose the details. I knew there was a reason I did my catechism study this morning! I sat down to do it before bed and realized I was already done for today and with joy found that my extra time could be in prayer with Randy. And it worked.

So, this is what transpired, and I wrote it down as quickly as I could.

Your mom loves you so much. And misses you so much. Please continue to guide them and watch over them. I know that you will because you do. And they know it, too but your signs are helpful to them.

He is so proud of what you are doing. It shows your continued love for him.

We/he gave you a big hug. You are in your bedroom. He holds you very close. We notice you have a hole in your heart. "It's broken," he says. He shows me that he has a mark there too. Your holes are almost matching. But his is more like a scar and yours is still hurting like an open wound. He tells me that his is fixed because Jesus healed him.

I remember back to when I first learned that he had died, and I saw the image of Mary cradling him in her arms. (I'm sorry about this next part, if it's hard, Heather). At first it was like she was holding a lifeless body after being shot. But then he was "consoled" back to life by her love and comfort and she gave him to Jesus to fix.

He explains his hole filled up with Jesus and healed.

As we watch you in your room now, he asks Jesus to heal your broken heart like he healed Randy's.

As we watch HIS finger touches you. Right on the little green hole in your heart. Your chest fills with light and love and turns the most beautiful baby blue color, filling you with your son's love. And it all shrinks down to just the size of the hole. This reminds me of your butterfly necklace.

Sleep in peace my friend, wrapped in the warm memories of your son. Wake anew tomorrow. Maybe you will feel changed, hopefully, you will feel your heart has been touched. I know it will always be hard for you, but I pray that you have many more little God moments that might help a bit of the hurt. I know I am grateful to have shared in this with Randy.

With love,
Heidi

Tears of joy and gratitude streamed down my face as I read her email. I remember feeling my heartbeat change to the point of panic the night before and then suddenly stop. According to Heidi's email, her experience and my experience happened at the same time. I firmly believe that Jesus, Randy Michael, and Heidi divinely touched my heart and brought healing. In gratitude, I sent Heidi an email the next morning and explained what transpired as I lay in bed the night before. I closed with, "Since my heart was touched and healed last night by HIM, I am now asking and trusting in HIM to touch and heal Elena's sinuses, to remove the tumor, and to give her a path to health moving forward. GOD IS GOOD and WILL DO GOOD."

Amazingly, the next week, Elena had surgery. The surgeon was able to remove the tumor, clear the infection, and avoid doing a craniotomy. It was a 14-hour surgery performed entirely through Elena's nose. She was home two days later and back in dental school in less than three weeks. To me, it was a miracle, not possible without divine intervention. Jesus really can take care of it all. We just need to believe and trust.

Since losing Randy Michael, my worldview has been profoundly transformed. Matters that previously seemed to be of great importance, like material items, entertainment, fashion, or dinner venues, now appear trivial, almost inconsequential. I've learned that "things" hold little true value, and that connections with people and genuine love for one another matter most.

This shift, while freeing, also brings a weight of sorrow that marks a loss of innocence. Our daughters have come to understand this, too. We all realize that darkness exists, and evil is a stark reality. Despite this newfound awareness, we remain grateful for blessings that endure despite our tremendous loss.

My current perspective on the world is both sobering and uplifting. We have encountered tragic loss, unrelenting grief, and a dark shadow that will forever linger. Yet we are uplifted because within this darkness, we have been overwhelmed by an outpouring of love and prayers from our family, friends, and community. Though humanity may falter at times, we have encountered individuals who have shown care, concern, kindness, and a level of generosity that surpasses our wildest imaginations. And as you can see from this Epilogue, we have been given so many beautiful signs that Randy Michael is at peace and fully restored. And these aren't even all of them. Our daughters, friends, and family have experienced his continued presence in a multitude of other remarkable ways.

For many months, Randy Michael wandered as a lost soul. On that glorious Easter Sunday, April 4, 2021, he returned to Mass at the Good Shepherd Parish in Cherry Creek, Colorado. This is ironic because the Good Shepherd always finds the lost sheep. On July 13, he went to Confession and later shared with his dad and me the relief he felt at being unburdened by incessant apologies. In the quiet hours before his passing, Randy Michael searched images of Jesus online, a testament to his yearning for mercy and forgiveness amid despair. His faith remained steadfast.

Months after Randy Michael's passing, we were going through his childhood memorabilia. I didn't save a lot of the kids' schoolwork. However, I came across this saint report Randy Michael wrote while he was in second grade. (Again, what are the chances?) You can read an excerpt from Randy Michael's report on Saint Peter in Photo 11.

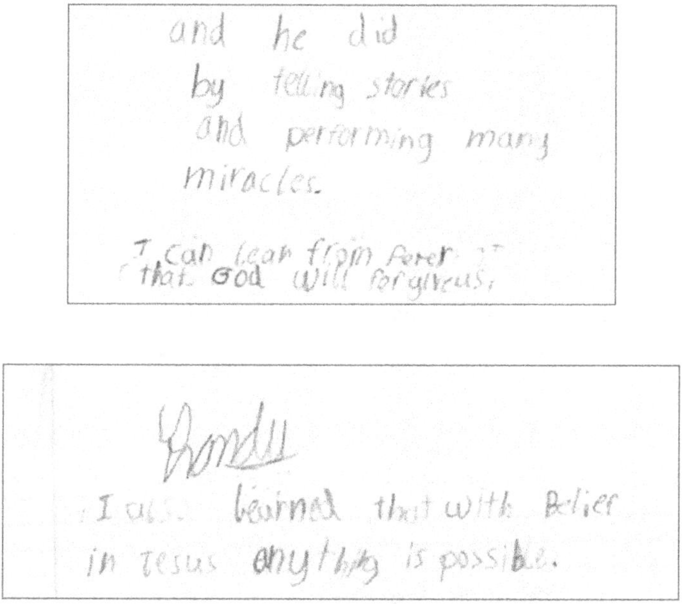

> and he did by telling stories and performing many miracles.
>
> I can learn from Peter that God will forgive us.

> Randy
>
> I also learned that with Belief in Jesus anything is possible.

Photo 11. Second-grade faith

Oh Jesus, I surrender myself to you, take care of everything.
—*The Sacred Heart of Jesus*

This was one more sign that gave us a sense of peace. We believe he returned home, resting in the trust of his Father's forgiveness, grace, love, and mercy. Randy Michael became a teacher in his absence. Through him, we have learned of God's kindness and mercy, and the enduring strength of his grace. Additionally, we have come to understand the inevitability of life's uncertainties, moments when our control falters.

We couldn't ultimately influence Randy Michael's choices. If we had been able to do that, this book would have remained unwritten. But what we can do is choose how we respond to this tragedy now. Our choice is to uphold our faith in God's plan and trust in him.

The journey following our son's tragic battle with cannabis-induced psychosis and the signs we've encountered since his passing have drawn us nearer to Jesus than ever before. We credit our son for this newly profound spiritual connection because of his actions right before he died and the signs that he has sent since that time.

Some days anger surges within us and we are dismayed by the ignorance of certain individuals and lawmakers and the societal permissiveness that allows companies to exploit addiction for profit. Yet, most days, we transform that anger and sadness into gratitude that we have learned the reasons behind our son's tragic fate. We're keenly aware that today's highly potent marijuana products were the root cause of our loss.

Now we channel our tragic experience into education, hoping to spare others from such heartache. We want everyone to embrace their individuality, to be extraordinary simply by being themselves. Everyone contributes a unique piece to the vast mosaic of humanity, creating a tapestry of diverse, personal narratives and gifts. Be Extraordinary, Be You.

So that is our love story, manifested in so many ways.

THE MYSTERY

The all-seeing Eye of God wept blind tears into my heart;
The all-powerful Voice of God spoke in silence to my heart;
The all-effulgent Light of God spread darkness in my heart.
In my blindness, I perceived;
Unhearing, I was attentive;
In darkness, I sought.
And seeking I was found; Darkness became my light;
Silence, a universal sound; Blindness, the watchful eye.
I continue searching –
And yet I am always found—
O mystery!

— Sr. Catherine Jenkins
1923–2021
(Randy Michael's Great, Great Aunt)

SIGNS OF CANNABIS USE:

1. Change in Behavior: Teens who use marijuana might seem more relaxed, but they can also become more forgetful, lazy, or have trouble focusing. You may notice that their motivation to do schoolwork or activities drops.

2. Red Eyes or Dry Mouth: As a vasodilator, a common physical sign is red or bloodshot eyes. Teens may also complain about having a dry mouth and drink more water than usual.

3. Smell on Clothes or Breath: Marijuana has a distinct smell, which can cling to teen's clothes, breath, room and even their car, however, vaped marijuana, whether in oil or solid form, often has little or no smell.

4. Sudden Mood Changes: A teen using marijuana might experience frequent mood swings, ranging from giggly and happy to irritable or erratic, and use can trigger anxiety and depression.

5. Changes in Eating Habits: Marijuana can increase appetite, so some teens may start eating more than usual, especially snacks or junk food (this is often referred to as "the munchies").

6. New Friend Groups or Isolation: You might notice a teen distancing themselves from old friends or hanging out with new people who may have a different influence on their behavior.

7. Decline in School Performance: Using marijuana can make it harder for teens to concentrate and remember things, which might lead to lower grades or skipping school.

8. Paranoia: Marijuana can cause psychosis, paranoia, schizophrenia, and suicidal tendencies and thoughts, especially if the child didn't previously show these symptoms.

9. Paraphernalia: Finding things like rolling papers, pipes, or vape pens may indicate marijuana use. Some teens may also use eye drops to reduce red eyes or burn incense to hide the smell.

SIGNS OF SUICIDAL BEHAVIOR

Behavioral Signs:

- Withdrawing from social connections – Isolation from family, friends, or activities.

- Increased use of drugs or alcohol – A marked rise in substance abuse.

- Giving away possessions – A sudden interest in distributing personal belongings.

- Saying goodbye – Expressing farewells to loved ones or writing goodbye letters.

- Risky or reckless behavior – Engaging in dangerous activities without concern for consequences.

- Sudden calmness – After a period of depression, a sudden shift to calm can indicate a decision has been made.

- Drastic changes in mood – Extreme mood swings, from sadness to irritability or agitation.

- Talking or writing about death – Open conversations or expressions about wanting to die.

- Loss of interest in activities – No longer caring about things once enjoyed.

Emotional Signs:

- Hopelessness – Feeling as though there's no future or solution to their problems.

- Despair – Talking about feeling trapped, in unbearable pain, or being a burden to others.

- Shame or guilt – Overwhelming feelings of being a failure or letting others down.

- Agitation or anxiety – Increased restlessness, panic, or worry about the future.

- Deep sadness or depression – Persistent and unshakable sadness or numbness.

- Verbal Cues: "I wish I were dead." "I can't go on anymore." "Everyone would be better off without me." "There's no reason to live."

Physical Changes:

- Neglecting personal appearance – A significant decline in grooming or hygiene.

- Disturbed sleep patterns – Sleeping too little, too much, or experiencing insomnia.

- Changes in eating habits – Noticeable weight loss or gain, or loss of appetite.

*Recognizing these signs is vital for taking action, seeking help, and potentially saving a life. If you notice these signs in someone, it's crucial to reach out and offer support. The National Suicide Prevention Lifeline is available by dialing "988," which connects individuals to immediate assistance and access to local resources for ongoing support.

ACKNOWLEDGMENTS

╰─╮

I wrote this book in honor and memory of our beloved son, Randy Michael Bacchus III. Although he was my greatest parenting challenge, he has also been my greatest teacher, helping me grow in ways I never imagined possible. I am blessed that he deepened my faith and trust in my higher power, Jesus. The various signs we've received, and Randy's own faith have been eye-opening. Randy taught me that no one is entirely good or entirely bad. Every human is a mix of both, and we must believe in God's forgiveness, grace, and mercy, and love one another no matter the circumstances.

Initially, I wrote a version of this book to remember his story and hold onto a piece of him. But as his story evolved, I learned vital information that needed to be shared with others. With the help of many, I hope that this book will educate others and prevent further tragedies within families and communities, as no one is immune to the grip of this widely accepted drug. I once despised public speaking, but now I dream of standing before audiences to share what I've learned, so others don't have to suffer.

I want to express my immense gratitude and respect to my husband, Randy Bacchus, who has endured more loss than any one person should bear, including the loss of his only son. The pain of losing a child is immeasurable and indescribable, leaving a hole that will never be filled. Yet, Randy has been a beacon of strength and resilience teaching me that, despite the tragedy we've faced, life goes on, and joy can still be found. His unwavering support has been vital in helping me share Randy Michael's story. From creating our website, filing for our nonprofit, and editing videos and presentations, Randy has been our business and marketing guru. I am forever grateful for his love and support, numerous talents, our shared faith, and his commitment to our family.

Our three beautiful daughters—Brooke, Sabrina, and Anna—light up our lives, and we are incredibly proud of their resilience, grit, and tenacity. Brooke, our eldest, was the last to see our handsome son and I cherish her decision to spend time with him on July 5th of 2021. One of her many strengths is now sharing his story, educating others, and supporting Be Extraordinary, Be You as a board member. Sabrina returned to college as a sophomore just a month after losing her beloved brother, and she recently graduated (on time, nonetheless). She now works as a Registered Nurse, and witnesses daily how addiction impacts so many of her patients. Anna was a rising high school junior when Randy Michael passed. Despite living with two grieving parents, she managed to bring love, laughter, and joy into our heavy home every day. Her cooking and hugs brought us jewels of comfort which was much needed. She is now a college sophomore and navigating a world where weed is normalized and considered "no big deal." These girls are our "why"—our reason to keep going.

I am grateful to countless family members and friends—far too many to name—who stood by us during our darkest days. Immediately in our hour of need, they brought meals, offered wisdom, prayed for us, and sent handwritten cards, texts, and phone calls to check in. Our community rallied around us during those initial days and months, and they continue to support us today. I hope you all know who you are. And thank you from the bottom of my heart.

Special thanks go to Randy Michael's true friends: Greta, Alec, and Olivia. They looked out for him, cared enough to set boundaries with him, and stood by him during his hardest moments. They also reached out to us when they saw he was suffering. Genuine friends are not afraid to speak up, and these friends truly loved our son.

I also want to thank those with special gifts who shared messages from our son: Jenni, Vincent, Anne, and Phoenix. Those messages and signs brought light to my darkest days.

In October 2021, our dear friend Maria handed me a copy of an article in *People* magazine that changed my life. Inside was an article about another mother who lost her son to cannabis-induced psychosis and suicide. As I read it, I was astonished by the similarities between our two boys and their families. At that moment, I understood the "why" behind what happened to our beautiful boy. I am forever grateful to that mother, Laura Stack, for sharing her story and turning her grief into prevention education.

I would also like to acknowledge our involvement with Smart Approaches to Marijuana (SAM and SAMMN). This incredible team of intelligent, caring individuals helped us testify in front of legislators regarding cannabis legalization in Minnesota. Even though our warnings fell on deaf ears, we felt empowered knowing we had done our part. Additionally, through the Parent Action Network (PAN), we were trained to write testimony and engage with the media. Together with SAM and PAN, we helped create Randy's Resolution in Congress alongside Congressman

Pete Sessions and Senator Pete Ricketts. This resolution calls for research, education, and policy development around high-potency marijuana.

In terms of writing this book, I owe a great debt of gratitude to those who helped with the development, editing, and refining: Jenny Schuna, Lynn Bartol, Ken Winters, Tammy Dittmore, Bob Land, Asya Blue, Luke Niforatos, and Crissy Groenewegen. They helped me clarify and expand on important details, making this book worth publishing.

Finally, I must thank our son. He left us in an instant with a million unanswered questions. But he also gave us many unanticipated gifts: video footage, journal entries, voicemails, and access to his records and documentation. He left us all the pieces to his puzzle, and we were able to put together the whole picture, which brought us peace and fueled our determination to share his story.

INDEX

Adderall, 115, 137, 139–40
addiction
    linked to higher THC levels, 31
    to marijuana, 65–66
    as pediatric-onset disorder, 27
    toll of, 20
    treatment for, 42
addiction prevention education, 186–87
ADHD. *See* attention deficit hyperactivity disorder
adolescence, brain development during, 178–79
Al-Anon, 190
amygdala, 179
anandamide, 176–77
anxiety, 43, 57, 94, 136, 179
apoptosis, 178
apple pipe, 40
Association of Recovery Schools, 43
attention deficit hyperactivity disorder, 15, 17, 43, 60, 136, 137
autism, 57

Bacchus, Anna, 11, 14, 29, 144–45, 147
Bacchus, Brooke, 11, 13, 49, 83, 86, 144–46, 150, 152, 195
Bacchus, Randy, 9–12, 36, 41–42, 63, 86–87, 90, 117, 119–22, 125, 129, 135, 141–42, 149, 151, 152, 156, 159, 173, 206
Bacchus, Randy Michael, 11
    adolescence of, 19–20
    aggressive behavior of, 55–57, 76–77, 127–29
    alcohol use by, 54–55
    autopsy of, 170
    at boarding school, 48–53
    caught using at home, 39–41
    clothing business of, 91, 97, 124, 138–39, 163, 204–5
    college planning for, 46–47, 51, 61, 67–68
    communications from, after his death, 211–15
    court records of, 105
    during COVID, 83–87, 91
    dealing with friend's suicide, 29–30

death of, 5, 149–51, 153–54, 156, 195–96
detox of, 121–24, 140
diagnoses for, 15, 39, 43–44, 57–59, 131, 136–37
drawings by, 196, 197, 201
early years of, 13–17
education of, 15–19, 44, 45, 48–54, 60–61, 81
employment of, 66, 68, 97, 99, 102–4, 133–37, 142, 146, 166
eulogy for, 162–71, 202
evaluations of, 14–17, 43–44, 115, 128, 134
faith of, 97, 102, 156, 160, 169, 216, 217
final days of, 159–60
financial management of, 134
in Florida for treatment, 121–25
gap year for, 61, 66
grandiose thinking of, 166–67
guns and, 128, 129, 130
hands of, 154, 156–57, 158, 196–98
hospitalization of, 115–16, 140
isolation of, 111–12
last days of, 159–60, 167
last visit with author, 95–96
law enforcement and, 36, 41, 56, 150–51

early marijuana use of, 20, 26–27
at MDA camp, 32–33
medical debts of, 140–41, 146
moving from Boulder to Denver, 108–9
moving to Colorado, 63
moving out, 45–46
musical aspirations of, 103, 110, 135, 139–40, 142, 143, 146, 148–49
paranoia of, 91, 95, 98, 102, 109, 112–14, 116, 119–20, 138, 141
psychotic episodes of, 68–69, 112–16, 119
referencing past traumas, 110–11
relocations of, 45–46, 61, 63
selling marijuana, 107, 126
signs from, 154–55, 159, 194–98, 202–7, 209, 210–11
suicidal ideations of, 69, 70, 71, 93, 130–31, 189
threatening self-harm, 125
toxicology report, final, 170
viewing of, 155–58, 196–98
visitation and funeral for, 161–66
web design business of, 91, 116, 124, 135
at wilderness camp, 119
writings of, 53, 69–72, 82, 84–87, 89–91, 97–98, 102,

135, 144, 148–50, 160, 166, 189, 196–201, 217
Bacchus, Sabrina, 11, 14, 47, 144–45, 152, 163
Bacchus family, 6–14, 20, 37–39, 42, 47, 55–57, 75–76, 90–91, 128, 144–45, 152–59, 186, 195–96, 216–18
Baker Act (Florida Mental Health Act of 1971), 125, 189
basal ganglia, 179
bat phone, 127–28, 128, 134–35
Be Extraordinary, Be You, 191, 204
bipolar disorder, 123, 136
blunt, 22
Blunt, James, 154
boarding school, therapeutic, 43, 48–52
bong, 24
brain
  development of, 177–80
  marijuana's effect on, 94, 131, 176–80
brain damage, 122
butterflies, 194–95, 198, 204–7

cannabidiol, 21–22, 174–75
cannabinoid 1, 176–77, 179–80
cannabinoid 2, 176, 177
cannabinoids, 21, 174

cannabis
  properties of, 174
  states' normalization of, 7
  tolerance breaks from, 81–82
  types of, 21
  US high school seniors' use of, 47
  See also marijuana
cannabis hyperemesis syndrome, 50–51, 64, 110
cannabis-induced psychosis, 69, 72, 73, 81, 92, 94, 98, 103, 115–16, 122–23, 131, 141, 159, 167–69, 180, 181
cannabis use disorder, 37, 39, 41, 44, 52, 59, 181
CBD. *See* cannabidiol
CB1. *See* cannabinoid 1
CB2. *See* cannabinoid 2
childhood seizure disorders, CBD prescribed for, 21, 174–75
Christian Health Share, 140
CHS. *See* cannabis hyperemesis syndrome
cognition, 94
cognitive functioning, impaired, 59, 92, 179
Colorado
  marijuana legalization in, 38, 56, 64, 105, 131, 182
  medical marijuana in, 127
  suicides in, 56, 182

Colorado Department of Public Health and Environment, 129
concentrates, 22
Concerta, 15, 16, 60
cool moms (parents), 26–27, 36, 187
court records, accessing, 105–6
COVID-19, 83–87, 91, 101, 112, 116, 134
CUD. *See* cannabis use disorder

dabbing (dabs), 23, 61
decision-making, deficits in, 59, 98, 178, 179
Delta-8, 21, 175
Delta-9, 175, 176. *See also* tetrahydrocannabinol
Delta-10, 21, 175
depersonalization, 72
depression, 43, 44, 57, 58, 94, 136
derived psychoactive cannabis products, 175
disruptive behavior disorders, 44
dopamine, 94, 177
DPCPs. *See* derived psychoactive cannabis products
drug prevention education, 186–87
drug testing, 45, 60, 185

drug use, discussing with children, 184–85, 187
dual-diagnosis treatment centers, 120–24, 190
dysgraphia, 16
dyslexia, 16
dysthymia, 58

edibles, 24–25, 175
educational outcomes, cannabis use and, 44
11-hydroxy-THC, 25
endocannabinoids, 174, 176–77
Epidiolex, 21, 174–75
executive functioning, reduced, 16, 17, 43, 59, 179

"Fall on Me" (Maverick City Music), 212
family contracts, 45
family mission statement, 186
family therapy, 128, 141–42
Farm Bill (Agriculture Improvement Act of 2018), 175
Fleet Farm General Store, 54
flower, 22–23
forgiveness, 193–94
420, 31
420 Day, 30, 61
Friedman, Russell, 193–94

Good Shepherd Parish (Cherry Creek , CO), 164, 216
gooning, 41
Grief Recovery Method, 193–94

hallucinations, auditory, 115, 116
heart problems, marijuana use and, 171
hemp, 21, 174–75
hemp-derived psychoactive cannabinoids, 21
Higher Power, learning on, 190–91
hippocampus, 179
hyperphagia, 179
hyperspirituality, 169
hypothalamus, 179

indica, 21, 174
involuntary commitment, 123
IQ, cannabis use and, 52
isolation, 112

James, John W., 193–94
Jenkins, Catherine, 219
Johnny's Ambassadors, 167
joint, 22

lawmaking, parents' engagement with, 188

Lev, Rohnet, 64
Life 360, 101, 107
local control, 188
LSD, 107

Mar-Anon, 190
Marbury, Chris, 156, 157–58, 160
Marchman Act (Florida), 123, 125, 189
marijuana
  addiction to, 65–67, 77, 170
  driving and, 38, 105
  effects on the brain, 94, 131, 176–80
  as foundation/gateway/promoter drug, 103
  isolation and, 112
  linked to other substance use, 103
  as medicine, 6
  potency of, 7, 21, 22, 31, 56, 59, 80, 173, 175–76, 180–82
  product types, potency of, 175–76
  reclassification of, 183
  selling of, 107
  signs of use, 188–89, 221–22
  sleep and, 137
  violent behavior and, 109
  ways to consume, 22–25
  withdrawal from, 65–67, 77, 170

See also cannabis
marijuana industry, 26
Maverick City Music, 212
MCRO. *See* Minnesota Court Records Online
medical marijuana, 107, 127
medical release of information, 58, 189
medications, vetting, 140
memorization capacity, 16, 17
mental health treatment options, awareness of, 189
micro dosing, 106–7
Miller, Mac, 104
Minnesota, marijuana legalization in, 173, 188
Minnesota Court Records Online, 105
mood disorder, 136
munchies, 179
Muscular Dystrophy Association camp, 32–33
mushrooms, psychoactive, 93, 106–7, 130
myelination, 178
myocardial infarction, marijuana use and, 171
"Mystery, The" (Jenkins), 219

Narcotics Anonymous, 190
National Institute on Drug Abuse, 103
National Suicide Prevention Lifeline, 225

neocortex, 179

oppositional defiant disorder, 43

paranoia, 94, 179
parents, advice for, 184–91
pipe, 23
posttraumatic stress disorder, 136, 141
pot propaganda, 26
prefrontal cortex, 59, 98, 178, 179
professional treatment, seeking, 190
psilocybin. *See* mushrooms, psychoactive
psychosis, 68, 72, 94, 136. *See also* cannabis-induced psychosis
PTSD. *See* posttraumatic stress disorder

Rocky Mountain High Intensity Drug Trafficking Area (HIDTA) Investigative Support Center, 38
roses, 195–96, 202–4, 207

Sabet, Kevin, 7
Saint Mary of the Lake Catholic Church (White Bear Lake, MN), 161
sativa, 21, 174
schizophrenia, 94, 123

cannabis use and, 72–73
marijuana potency and, 180–81
scrommiting, 64. *See also* cannabis hyperemesis syndrome
self-harm, threats of, 125
710 Day, 61
Stack, Laura, 167
sleep, 137
Smart Approaches to Marijuana, Minnesota, 173
smokable flower, 22–23
sober high school and colleges, 43
Stack, John, 167
Stack, Johnny, 167
steam showers, 50–51
stroke, marijuana use and, 171
Substance Abuse and Mental Health Services Administration, 128
substance-use disorder, 27
suicidal behavior, signs of, 223–25
suicidal ideation, 56, 57, 131, 181–82
suicide, aftermath of, 5–6, 28–30, 32, 79
support groups, 190
synaptogenesis, 178

THC (tetrahydrocannabinol), 21–22, 174, 175
age of first use, significance of, 180
edibles, 24–25
endocannabinoids and, 176–77
frequency of use, 180
mental health and, 180–82
stored in fat cells, 66
suicidal ideation and, 181–82
testing for, 60
THC-O, 21, 175
THC-P, 21, 175
THCV, 175
therapists, vetting, 47
Things They Don't Teach You in School (Dingee), 134
three-way calls, medical billing and, 141
tic disorder, 14–15
tolerance break, 81–82

United States
daily marijuana use in, 31
legal status of cannabis in, 7
U.S. Drug Enforcement Administration, 183
U.S. Food and Drug Administration, 21, 174–75
vaping, 23–24, 65, 80, 175, 184

Vyvanse, 115

Washington state, marijuana
 legalization in, 105
water pipe, 24
wellness checks, 113, 125, 127,
 150–52
what-ifs, 193–94
wilderness camp, 32, 41–43

"You're Beautiful" (Blunt),
 154

www.ingramcontent.com/pod-product-compliance
Lightning Source LLC
Chambersburg PA
CBHW020537030426
42337CB00013B/885